The AIDS Health Crisis

Psychological and Social Interventions

APPLIED CLINICAL PSYCHOLOGY

Series Editors:
Alan S. Bellack, *Medical College of Pennsylvania at EPPI, Philadelphia, Pennsylvania,* and Michel Hersen, *University of Pittsburgh, Pittsburgh, Pennsylvania*

A Continuation Order Plan is available for this series. A continuation order will bring delivery of each new volume immediately upon publication. Volumes are billed only upon actual shipment. For further information please contact the publisher.

The AIDS Health Crisis

Psychological and Social Interventions

Jeffrey A. Kelly

University of Mississippi Medical Center
Jackson, Mississippi

and

Janet S. St. Lawrence

Jackson State University and
University of Mississippi Medical Center
Jackson, Mississippi

Plenum Press • New York and London

Library of Congress Cataloging in Publication Data

Kelly, Jeffrey A.
  The AIDS health crisis.

  (Applied clinical psychology)
  Bibliography: p.
  Includes index.
  1. AIDS (Disease)—Psychological aspects. 2. AIDS (Disease)—Social aspects. 3. AIDS
(Disease)—Patients—Rehabilitation. I. St. Lawrence, Janet S. II. Title. III. Series.
[DNLM: 1. Acquired Immunodeficiency Syndrome—prevention & control. 2. Ac-
quired Immunodeficiency Syndrome—psychology. 3. Psychology, Social. WD 308
K29a]
RC607.A26K45   1988   362.1′969792   88-17881

ISBN-13: 978-1-4612-8287-7   e-ISBN-13: 978-1-4613-1003-7
DOI: 10.1007/978-1-4613-1003-7

First Printing—September 1988
Second Printing—September 1989

© 1988 Plenum Press, New York
 Softcover reprint of the hardcover 1st edition 1988
A Division of Plenum Publishing Corporation
233 Spring Street, New York, N.Y. 10013

To the dedicated professionals on the front
lines of the health crisis who compassionately care
for persons with AIDS

Preface

Acquired immune deficiency syndrome (AIDS) poses a health threat unparalleled in modern times. Identified just a few years ago, AIDS and the human immunodeficiency virus (HIV) responsible for it affect millions of persons worldwide. AIDS has already become the leading cause of death among persons under 40 in some large American cities.

From the beginning, it has been evident that AIDS carries unique psychological and social ramifications. In spite of its lethality, new cases of HIV infection are preventable if individuals can be assisted to make behavior changes to lessen or eliminate viral transmission. To the extent that we can develop effective primary prevention interventions, it will be possible to keep larger numbers of people from becoming infected with the HIV virus. Psychological and social risk-behavior change interventions, whether at the level of individual clients, groups, or entire communities, can play a key role—in fact, the only available role—in disease prevention.

Patients with any life-threatening illness have psychological, social, and support needs. However, these needs are more pronounced and, often, less easily addressed for persons affected by AIDS. People in good clinical health but with HIV infection face years of worry concerning whether they will develop AIDS. Nearly 2 million Americans are currently in this precarious position; by 1991, 50 to 100 million persons worldwide are expected to share the same uncertainty. People with HIV illnesses other than AIDS, the hundreds of thousands with so-called "AIDS-related complex" diseases, must cope not only with fear of AIDS but also with symptoms that provide physical evidence that their immune system functioning is already impaired. Patients with the most serious diseases caused by HIV infection—those with AIDS itself—face the probability of debilitation and death within several years of diagnosis. Not surprisingly, the mental health and social needs of these groups are great.

Unfortunately, persons with AIDS, AIDS-related illnesses, and even asymptomatic HIV infection often have few resources available to them in their long and difficult coping process. Because of the widespread hysteria that surrounds AIDS, persons affected by HIV may face ostracism, avoidance, and fear by their families, friends, loved ones, and even some health care providers. Depression, anxiety, anger, and feelings of helplessness—common responses to any life-threatening illness, are even more common for an illness that is usually acquired sexually or through drug use. In part because of widespread public misunderstandings about AIDS and in part because most AIDS patients are members of groups that were viewed negatively even before the health crisis began, persons with AIDS fear—and often face—discrimination, stigma, and punitive social responses.

This book is written for psychologists, social workers, nurses, physicians, counselors, and others who work with AIDS patients or persons at risk for AIDS. Just as AIDS is a new health threat to society, it also represents a new area for mental health, community intervention, and social service professionals. Few of us were ever trained to deal with the problems experienced by persons with AIDS, and few professionals were specifically trained in areas essential to the prevention of this disease. Yet the growing crisis means that help providers in many disciplines and in all areas of the country will inevitably see ever-larger numbers of people threatened or already affected by AIDS.

The aims of this book are to familiarize mental health, social service, and counseling professionals in practice or in training with information about AIDS and its risk behaviors; to review behavior-change methods for the primary prevention of HIV infection for individual clients, for groups, or at a community level; to discuss psychological and social difficulties experienced by persons with AIDS and HIV infection; and to outline clinical interventions that can help to alleviate some of these difficulties. Because AIDS was so recently identified, prevention and psychological/social treatment intervention strategies have only recently been studied. Where gaps in research on prevention and intervention exist—and there are clearly many gaps—the authors have attempted to incorporate strategies from other areas of the behavior-change/prevention, behavioral medicine, and illness-coping literature that are also relevant to AIDS. While this book is intended for practitioners, we have presented intervention strategies that are substantiated by empirical research findings.

Much of the literature described in this book involves prevention and clinical interventions for homosexual men or intravenous drug users who have AIDS or who are at risk for AIDS. There are two reasons for this focus. One is that the majority of present American AIDS patients are gay or bisexual men or intravenous drug users. As a result, clinical interventions will often be for persons in these groups. The second reason is that most behavioral research, especially in the prevention area, has been conducted in the gay community and, to a lesser degree, with intravenous drug users. The lessons learned from interventions with these groups will no doubt prove relevant to other populations as well, including adults who may become exposed to HIV infection through heterosexual contacts. The psychosocial difficulties of young children with AIDS are substantial, but they often differ from those of adults and are not the primary focus of attention.

Parts of this book may be perceived by some as controversial. We doubt that it is possible for any book, or for any intervention or service program relating to AIDS, to be without some potential for controversy. That is the nature of the topic. However, we have always attempted to anchor the book's content in sound science, sound practice, and ethical and compassionate treatment for persons who are threatened or affected by the disease.

New developments in AIDS research occur quickly. Some of these developments involve better understanding of the immunological processes related to HIV infection, while others involve advances in medical treatment, epidemiology, prevention, and service provision. The authors have incorporated the most recent and up-to-date information available at the time this book was prepared. As research in this area advances, new and revised conclusions may need to be reached.

We are indebted to a number of persons who assisted in the book's development. Teddy L. Brasfield and Harold V. Hood contributed not only research assistance in preparing the book but also their valuable suggestions and critiques. Wauline Carter did a superb job preparing early and final drafts of the manuscript. Special thanks are also due to Eddie Sandifer and Hillary Chiz for making specialized background materials available to the authors.

Jeffrey A. Kelly
Janet S. St. Lawrence

Jackson, Mississippi

Contents

Medical Aspects of AIDS

In the spring of 1981, investigators at the UCLA Medical Center recorded five cases of *Pneumocystis carinii* pneumonia, a virulent form of pneumonia uncommon in the United States (Centers for Disease Control, 1981a). Within a few months, clinical researchers in New York, San Francisco, and Los Angeles discovered 25 cases of Kaposi's sarcoma, an exceedingly unusual cancer among young and otherwise healthy persons in this country (Centers for Disease Control, 1981b). None of the patients suffered from any underlying illness that would account for the development of these often fatal and unusual diseases, but each patient exhibited severe immune system impairment for unknown reasons and each was a young homosexual male. The syndrome accounting for these first few cases was not yet named but would shortly be identified as acquired immune deficiency syndrome (AIDS). Within just a few years, it would be considered the most serious infectious disease epidemic of modern times and be designated as the nation's primary medical priority by the National Institutes of Health.

Since AIDS was first identified, it has been the subject of intense medical and epidemiological research. In this chapter, we will review basic medical characteristics of the syndrome, examine trends and projections concerning its prevalence, and discuss issues related to the health course of AIDS-affected persons. While a great deal has been learned about AIDS over the past few years, much is still unknown and many

controversies still exist concerning medical aspects of AIDS. In this overview, we will present the findings that are consensually accepted by most
researchers, as well as medical hypotheses that are now well substantiated.

1.1. MEDICAL CHARACTERISTICS OF AIDS

For surveillance purposes, AIDS is defined as a reliably diagnosed
opportunistic disease or infection that is predictive of cellular immune
deficiency and occurs in a person with no known preexisting illnesses or
therapies that would produce immunosuppression (Groopman, et al.,
1985; Haverkos & Drotman, 1984; Jaffe, Bregman, & Selik, 1985). This
definition of AIDS entails three components: (1) identification of an opportunistic disease; (2) establishment of cellular immune deficiency, either by clinical laboratory tests or by the presence of a disease associated
with immunosuppression; and (3) ruling out alternative factors that
might cause immune deficiency, such as lymphoma, leukemia, congeni-
tal immunodeficiency, or a history of steroid or other immunosuppressive therapies. Because AIDS development hinges on compromised
immune system functioning, we will turn our attention first to the
origin of AIDS-related immune deficiency and then to its medical
consequences.

1.1.1. HIV and Its Relation to AIDS

When AIDS first appeared, severe immune system compromise was
quickly and consistently recognized in its victims, but the underlying
causes for the immune system failure were unknown. Within several
years, independent investigators in France and the United States identified unusual serum antibodies in a large majority of AIDS patients
(Barre-Sinoussi et al., 1983; Gallo et al., 1984; Montagnier et al., 1984;
Safai et al., 1984). The virus responsible for the antibodies was termed
lymphadenopathy-associated virus (LAV) by the French researchers and
human T-cell lymphotropic virus type III (HTLV-III) by the American
researchers. Later, it would be termed the human immunodeficiency
virus (HIV). All three designations refer to an identical retrovirus that
infects and attacks helper T lymphocytes, the cells that activate immune
system functioning.[*] Similar retroviruses had been isolated previously.
HTLV-II, for example, is often found in patients with T-cell leukemia,

where it produces immunosuppression (Blattner & Gallo, 1985). However, HIV's discovery and its identification as the virus responsible for AIDS set the stage for a better understanding of the disease as well as the methods by which it is transmitted.

The HIV virus is clinically identified and most often tracked by the presence of serum antibodies. The HIV antibody is commonly found, as one would expect, in patients with AIDS (Laurence *et al.*, 1984; Safai *et al.*, 1984). HIV antibodies are also present in patients who show some clinical symptoms of immune suppression but who do not have the clear-cut opportunistic infections characteristic of AIDS. For example, patients with persistent generalized lymphadenopathy, chronic enlargement of lymph nodes in multiple body sites unrelated to identifiable illness or infection and indicative of abnormal immune function, are also HIV antibody-positive 77 to 100% of the time (Bayer, Bienzle, Schneider, & Hunsmann, 1984; Lang *et al.*, 1987; Laurence *et al.*, 1984). Further, HIV serum antibodies are found among currently healthy individuals who have been exposed to the virus. Depending on the geographical area and the behavioral characteristics of subjects recruited for research participation, HIV-antibody-positive rates among sexually active but apparently healthy homosexual males range from 20 to 60% in many locations (Anderson & Levy, 1985; Carlson *et al.*, 1985; Goedert *et al.*, 1984, 1985; Jaffe, Darrow *et al.*, 1985; Lang *et al.*, 1987). Other groups at risk for AIDS also exhibit higher than expected HIV seropositivity. These groups include intravenous drug users, hemophiliacs who received transfusions before programs to detect HIV-contaminated blood were instituted, heterosexual partners of persons with known HIV infection, and female prostitutes (Brettle *et al.*, 1986; Carlson *et al.*, 1985; Chamberlain *et al.*, 1984; *Journal of the American Medical Association*, 1987a; Harris *et al.*, 1983; Redfield *et al.*, 1987; Robert-Guroff *et al.*, 1986).

1.1.1.1. Consequences of HIV Exposure

Epidemiological research now indicates that a very large number of people, probably approaching 2 million in the United States, have been exposed to HIV and are antibody-positive (or seropositive) to it (Curran,

*From the time of its discovery, controversy has existed concerning the name of the virus, with French investigators terming it LAV and some American researchers favoring the term HTLV-III. The designation "human immunodeficiency virus" (HIV) was proposed by the International Committee for Taxonomy of Viruses (Centers for Disease Control, 1986b) and will be used in this text.

1985). From 50 to 100 million persons worldwide will be exposed by 1991 (World Health Organization, 1987). The proportion of persons who are exposed and antibody-positive to HIV and who are also actively carrying the virus is not conclusively known, but most HIV seropositive individuals are presumed to be infected (Centers for Disease Control, 1985a; Goedert et al., 1984; Melby et al., 1984). Because the majority of individuals antibody-positive to HIV are actually infected with the virus, persons with HIV antibodies are generally presumed to be carriers and, therefore, capable of transmitting the virus to others even when they show no evidence of illness.

A key question with respect to AIDS epidemiology involves the health course of people who become infected by HIV. Unfortunately, and in spite of vigorous investigation, this is an aspect of AIDS research where definitive conclusions have proven elusive. Long-term consequences of HIV infection are difficult to predict because the clinical manifestations of the virus vary across individuals, AIDS is newly discovered, most major longitudinal prospective studies of HIV-exposed persons have not yet been completed, and behavioral, constitutional, and other risk cofactors may influence the future health course of individual patients. Difficulties predicting the health course of HIV-exposed persons are exacerbated by the potentially long incubation period of the virus. The latency from initial virus exposure to clinical disease onset appears to range from 1 year to as many as 14 years (Groopman, 1985; Peterman et al., 1985; Seale, 1985).

In spite of these health prediction obstacles, a consensus has emerged among most AIDS investigators that from among the large population of HIV-infected persons, a proportion will eventually develop AIDS. Current studies suggest that from 5 to 20% of virus carriers will succumb to the disease in its full clinical criterion form within 5 years of infection (Curran, 1985; Eyster et al., 1985; Francis & Petriccian, 1985; Groopman, 1985; Hessol et al., 1987). An additional, and probably larger, proportion of HIV carriers will develop symptoms of immune system compromise, show some clinical signs of illness, but not immediately exhibit diagnosable and clear-cut evidence of opportunistic disease. The most common of these HIV-infection disorders is persistent generalized lymphadenopathy, although a variety of HIV-related diseases, ranging from mild to more serious, have been consolidated in imprecise fashion under the diagnostic umbrella known as "AIDS-related complex" (ARC) disorders (Allen, 1984; Groopman, 1985; Volberding, 1984). Some patients deteriorate from ARC status to full-blown AIDS when they develop an opportunistic illness such as pneumocystic pneumonia, Kaposi's sarcoma, or one of the other benchmark diseases characterizing AIDS. However, other patients have only mild symptoms of immune insufficiency, which do not progress into full-blown AIDS, at least over the short term. Finally, many—and possibly most—persons who are currently antibody-positive to HIV are asymptomatic and show no detectable clinical evidence of either immune suppression or illness. Because AIDS has been researched for only a relatively brief period of time, it is not possible to predict the health course of these individuals years into the future. However, it is likely that some HIV antibody-positive persons remain asymptomatic and healthy while also remaining carriers and potential transmitters of the virus to others.

To summarize, a range of potential health consequences can follow exposure to the human immunodeficiency virus. The most serious is a clinical-criterion AIDS that develops in at least 5 to 20% of those infected with HIV within several years of virus exposure and develops in more patients later. A number of other transient or persistent conditions characteristic of immune insufficiency are present in an additional pro-portion of HIV-infected persons; these disorders, which range from mild to clinically significant in severity, may but do not invariably worsen in the short term. Other individuals, although exposed to the virus, develop no symptoms of disease and have no evidence of immune system compromise for at least several years following their exposure.

1.1.1.2. Determinants of Health Course

Since the disease outcomes of HIV exposure are variable, a question that naturally arises involves the determinants of an individual's specific health course. While there have been many hypotheses advanced to ad-dress this question, definitive conclusions have not yet been reached. Attention usually focuses on the action of the virus and on the role of cofactors.

If the human immunodeficiency virus is the sole causal agent of AIDS and if an individual can become infected following one adequate expo-sure, the individual's health course could be determined simply by the length of time since HIV exposure and the natural speed with which the virus attacks critical cells in the immune system. Variable outcomes, ranging from asymptomatic carrier status to the development of mild or severe disease, are well known for certain other viral infections, such as hepatitis type-B, and HIV may operate in a similar manner.

On the other hand, the relationship between HIV exposure and health course may be mitigated by a variety of potential cofactors. For example, repeated reexposure to the virus or to its different strains following an initial exposure may increase the likelihood of immune system abnormality and the probability of full clinical disease onset. Some investigators have proposed that actual AIDS disease onset may be determined by an interaction between HIV and other infectious viruses that can also impair immune system function, such as the Epstein-Barr virus and cytomegalovirus (Ciobanu & Wiernik, 1986; Drew, 1986; Sonnabend, Witkin, & Purtilo, 1985). Attention has also been focused on whether genetic characteristics of the host may influence whether an HIV-infected person remains healthy, develops mild clinical symptoms of immunocompromise, or develops full-blown AIDS (Eales *et al.*, 1987). Some investigators have further speculated that the use of chemical substances that independently suppress immune function (including inhaled volatile nitrites or "poppers," excessive alcohol consumption, and other recreational drugs), the individual's general health and fitness, stress, and other psychological or behavioral factors may influence health course (see Coates, Stall, *et al.*, 1987; Goedert, 1985; Jaffe *et al.*, 1983; Landesman & Viera, 1983; Marmor *et al.*, 1982; Temoshok, Zich, Solomon, & Stites, 1987). Thus, while HIV has been established as the primary agent causing AIDS and HIV-related diseases, a variety of other behavioral and constitutional factors have been proposed, but not yet empirically confirmed, as possible comitigators of actual disease development.

1.1.1.3. Other Characteristics of HIV

When HIV becomes activated in a person, the virus binds to T-4 (or "helper T") lymphocytes of the immune system, causing them to lose their normal capacity to activate other immune system cells and to die prematurely. Another type of lymphocyte, termed T-8 (or "suppressor T") cells, deactivates certain immune responses. The ratio of T-4 to T-8 cells (or helper to suppressor T cells) or the absolute number of T cells are taken as indices of immune system integrity. In patients with AIDS and AIDS-related illnesses, the absolute number of circulating helper T cells and the ratio of helper to suppressor cells are frequently reduced (Boyko *et al.*, 1985; Groopman, Sarngadharan *et al.*, 1985). Thus, on a simplified cellular level, HIV incapacitates and destroys the lymphocytes that activate the immune system, leaving intact those cells that decelerate immune system response. The clinical consequence is immunosuppression and a diminished ability to respond to diseases against which the body could normally defend itself. Reductions of T-4 cells or a reduced T-4:T-8 cell ratio predict deterioration in the clinical health of persons infected with the virus (Goedert *et al.*, 1987; Polk *et al.*, 1987). There is evidence that HIV eludes immune system attack by binding to helper T cells and there is additional evidence that multiple strains of the virus exist (Brun-Vezinet *et al.*, 1987; Gallo, 1987; Gibbons, Parks, Parks, Hahn, & Shaw, 1987). The origin of HIV is not conclusively known, although AIDS is highly prevalent and responsible for hundreds of thousands of deaths in areas of central Africa (Clumeck *et al.*, 1984; Clumeck, Van de Perre, Carael, Rouvroy, & Nzaramba, 1985).

In spite of its lethality, the human immunodeficiency virus is surprisingly delicate and is not transmissible except in specific and narrow ways. It is present in body fluids, especially blood and semen, and transmission of the virus from an infected to a noninfected person requires that HIV-infected fluids gain direct entry into the recipient's bloodstream. Unlike the airborne and highly contagious viruses responsible for illness such as colds and influenza, HIV is transmitted by blood-to-blood contact (such as would occur when drug abusers share needles, when a person is transfused with blood that is HIV-infected, when an infant is born to an HIV-infected mother, or by sexual activities in which an infected person's semen, blood, or body fluids can enter the partner's bloodstream (Centers for Disease Control, 1986a). As we will discuss in Chapter 2, the virus is not transmitted during the course of even close everyday social contact with an HIV-infected person.

1.1.1.4. Identification of HIV Antibody Status

Shortly after HIV was identified, laboratory tests were developed to detect the presence of viral antibodies in blood. The purpose of these tests was to screen blood bank donations in order to prevent the inadvertent administration of HIV-contaminated blood to transfusion recipients and, thus, to preserve the safety of blood bank supplies.

The test most commonly used to detect HIV serum antibodies employs the enzyme-linked immunosorbent assay (ELISA) technique. The test, commercially manufactured by several pharmaceutical laboratories, is highly sensitive to the presence of HIV antibodies, but it generates a

relatively large number of "false positive" results by erroneously desig-
nating blood samples as HIV antibody-positive when they are not, on the
basis of standard criteria for test result interpretation (see Carlson *et al.*,
1985; *Journal of the American Medical Association*, 1985). The rate of false
positives using the ELISA test depends on the actual prevalence of HIV
antibodies in the population providing the blood samples (*JAMA*, 1985),
as well as certain previous illnesses of the person providing the sample,
but the test generates few "false negatives." Therefore, it rarely designates a sample as free of HIV antibodies when they are actually present.
This, of course, is the sensitivity characteristic that is most desirable when
the purpose of the laboratory test is to screen out infected samples and
safeguard blood bank supplies. All major blood banks in the United
States and in most other countries now screen donated serum for antibodies.

The ELISA test for detecting HIV antibodies was originally developed to protect blood bank supplies and not to serve as a patient diagnostic measure. However, given interest in detecting the virus for clinical
purposes, the ELISA test is also used to evaluate serum samples from
patients and from persons seeking to learn their HIV antibody status.
When employed for these purposes, the ELISA screen is usually repeated
to obtain better reliability with respect to false positive results. But because the ELISA procedure, even with repeated testings, still has a tendency to label samples as antibody-positive when they are not, different
laboratory techniques are used for confirmation. The most common,
termed the Western blot test, is a more expensive and time-consuming
laboratory method for detecting HIV antibodies, is less sensitive than the
ELISA to their presence, but is also less likely to yield false positives
(Carlson *et al.*, 1985; *Journal of the American Medical Association*, 1985).
Thus, the Western blot test or an immunofluorescence assay functions to
rule out false positive ELISA findings and to establish the antibody's
actual presence; reactive results on both tests are taken as evidence confirming viral exposure.

While HIV antibody testing serves a useful clinical/diagnostic function in the evaluation of patients suspected of having AIDS, an AIDS-
related disease, or other evidence of immune system compromise, HIV
testing of healthy individuals is controversial. When ELISA results are
confirmed by the Western blot procedure, an individual can know
whether he or she has been exposed to HIV. If exposed, the individual

can take steps to prevent potential transmission of the virus to others and can seek regular medical attention to monitor his or her health status (Association of State and Territorial Health Officials Foundation, 1985; Hopkins, 1987a). On the other hand, concerns about the negative ramifications of wide-scale, nonvoluntary testing for apparently healthy persons have also been widely expressed (Bayer, Levine, & Wolf, 1986; Miller, Jeffries, Green, Harris, & Pinching, 1986). These concerns center on the fact that antibody screening confirms past exposure to the virus rather than current health or prognosis, that positive antibody status can cause great worry about one's future health course and lead to maladaptive coping, and that the identification of an individual as HIV-positive could easily result in discrimination with respect to education, employment, housing, insurance, and social stigma. In addition, it may require several months for a person exposed to HIV to develop detectable antibodies (Cooper *et al.*, 1985). Thus, negative antibody results, unless repeated several months apart with no interceding possibility of exposure, may not accurately reflect exposure status. There have also been cases of individuals who carry the virus but are antibody-negative even with repeated testing (Groopman, Hartzband, *et al.*, 1985; Mayer *et al.*, 1986). Most organizations advise apparently healthy members of AIDS risk groups to refrain from any activities that would allow the transmission of HIV from one person to another, regardless of whether an HIV-antibody test is taken. When voluntary antibody testing is sought, the "healthy but curious" individual is often advised to do so only under circumstances that assure anonymity and provide opportunities for follow-up counseling.

1.2. DISEASES RELATED TO HIV INFECTION

As noted earlier, HIV reduces the number of helper T lymphocytes and, in doing so, undermines the immune system's capacity to resist many infections and illnesses. Because immunocompromised persons are susceptible to an exceedingly wide range of bacterial, viral, fungal, and protozoan diseases, it is difficult to catalog all of the specific illnesses developed by these patients. Further, persons with immune suppression are often affected simultaneously by multiple opportunistic infections. In this section, we will first review those opportunistic diseases that are often associated with AIDS and then discuss the less clear-cut illnesses that occur in other HIV diseases.

TABLE 1
Diseases and Infections Commonly Associated with AIDS

	Malignancies
Kaposi's sarcoma	Lesions affecting the skin, oral mucosa, and visceral organs
Malignant lymphomas	Non-Hodgkin lymphoma most frequently affecting the central nervous system, bone marrow, and bowel
Oral, anorectal, and other malignancies	Although Kaposi's sarcoma and malignant lymphomas are the most common, increased incidence of other malignancies is also found with AIDS
	Protozoa
Pneumocystis carinii pneumonia	The most common opportunistic disease afflicting AIDS patients
Toxoplasma gondii	Commonly manifested clinically by encephalitis A small bowel organism producing cramps and diarrhea
	Viruses
Cytomegalovirus	Produces major organ dysfunction, often affecting gastrointestinal, adrenal, and vision systems
Herpes	Herpes simplex and zoster infections are unusually extensive and virulent in AIDS patients
Epstein-Barr virus	Produces fever, lymphadenopathy, fatigue, and other symptoms
	Fungi
Candida	Candida infections particularly affect mucus membranes of oral and digestive tract; respond to therapy but recur
Crytococcus neoformans	Commonly manifested clinically by meningitis
	Bacteria
Mycobacterium species	Several Mycobacterium species produce symptoms including fatigue, weight loss, and fever

1.2.1 Diseases Associated with AIDS (Table 1)

1.2.1.1. Pneumocystis carinii Pneumonia

Pneumocystic pneumonia, the most common life-threatening opportunistic disease associated with AIDS, is diagnosed in at least 60% of new AIDS patients (Centers for Disease Control, 1983), although it may be even more prevalent by the end stages of AIDS. Caused by the *P. carinii* bacterium and verified by laboratory tests identifying the organism in lung tissue or bronchial secretions, this infection has a mortality rate of up to 60% per acute episode (Kovacs & Masur, 1984), although early clinical trials with drugs such as azido-deoxythymidine (AZT) result in significantly lessened frequency and mortality of acute *P. carinii* episodes (Mitsuya et al., 1985; Yarchoan & Broder, 1987; Yarchoan et al., 1987). Early symptoms of the illness often include intermittent fever, chills, weight loss, cough and chest discomfort, or shortness of breath; the acute onset of the disease in AIDS patients often follows within 2 to 10 weeks of such symptoms (Macher & Reichert, 1984).

1.2.1.2. Kaposi's Sarcoma

Kaposi's sarcoma (KS), first identified in the late 1800s, is a disease that primarily afflicted elderly males of Jewish or Mediterranean descent and Africans. In these populations, Kaposi's sarcoma malignancies attracted little notice because of their very slow growth course and relatively uncommon occurrence. However, Kaposi's is prevalent among AIDS patients—affecting approximately 33% of all cases—and is also highly virulent and aggressive. Kaposi's sarcoma cooccurs with pneumocystic pneumonia in approximately 7% of AIDS patients. For reasons that are not yet well understood, Kaposi's sarcoma is considerably more prevalent among homosexual AIDS patients than among AIDS patients from other risk groups (Centers for Disease Control, 1981b). Kaposi's sarcoma usually first appears as red, purple, or blue palpable, nonpainful cutaneous tumors that occur in any body area. They often increase in number and are frequently accompanied by lymph node enlargement, fever, weight loss, and night sweats (Volberding, 1984). Effective treatments for the malignancy have not yet been developed, in part because many drugs that might retard Kaposi's sarcoma are themselves immunosuppressing. AIDS patients with Kaposi's sarcoma do not usually die from that malignancy *per se*, but rather from other opportunistic infections that cooccur with KS in AIDS patients (Volberding, 1984).

1.2.1.3 . Other Infections

A variety of other diseases are associated with AIDS and may exist concurrently with both pneumocystic pneumonia and Kaposi's sarcoma. *Candida* infections ("thrush") are fungal in nature and primarily affect the oral cavity, esophagus, and rectum. Oral candida is evidenced by sore

throat or mouth, low-grade fever, pain when swallowing, or mouth ul-
cers. Although treatable with antifungal agents, candida episodes recur
in many immunocompromised patients. *Cryptococcus* infections, also a
fungal disease, and *toxoplasmosis*, a protozoan infection, can each affect
the central nervous system, producing meningitis, encephalitis, and a
variety of serious concomitant central nervous system/neurological
problems. *Herpes simplex* infections are common in patients with AIDS
and are much more extensive, virulent, and recurrent among immunocompromised individuals than in persons with immune system integrity.
The ulcerative lesions most frequently occur in the oral, esophageal, and
perirectal areas. *Cytomegalovirus* is a virus common in the general population, where it usually remains latent. In immunocompromised patients
with AIDS, the virus proliferates rapidly and is often characterized by
such symptoms as fever, weight loss, diarrhea, and severe malaise. Cytomegalovirus infections ultimately produce major dysfunction affecting
the lungs, gastrointestinal tract, and other organ systems. There is no
effective treatment for acute cytomegalovirus infection, and severe disease contributes to the deaths of a significant proportion of AIDS patients.

Although these infections are among the most common in AIDS patients, dozens more opportunistic diseases have also been diagnosed.
They include malignant neoplasms other than Kaposi's sarcoma (affecting the central nervous system, bone marrow, and other sites) and an
array of bacterial, viral, fungal, and protozoan infections.* These are not
"new" diseases, and all are known to occur in persons without AIDS.
However, the immune deficiency characterizing AIDS makes these diseases more common in persons who would not ordinarily be expected to
have them and makes these infections more extensive, aggressive, recurrent, and life threatening to an AIDS patient. The HIV virus is also
capable of directly affecting a number of organ systems and the central
nervous system. CNS involvement occurs frequently in AIDS patients,
and a large number of patients exhibit evidence of memory loss, dementia, organic brain syndrome, and other motor or sensory nervous system
impairment, especially in late stages of the illness (Ho *et al.*, 1986; Lowenstein & Sharfstein, 1983; Wolcott, 1986a).

---

* A detailed discussion of the full symptoms, clinical consequences, and medical treatments
for the many opportunistic infections associated with AIDS and HIV infection is beyond the
scope of this book. The reader may wish to consult such volumes as DeVita, Hellman, and
Rosenberg (1985), Ebbesen, Biggar, and Melbye (1984), or Staquet, Hemmen, and Baert
(1986) for a more detailed review of these topics.

Over the course of their disease, most AIDS patients experience a long series of increasingly debilitating infections. Depending on the stage when AIDS is first diagnosed, mortality exceeds 80% 2 years following the diagnosis, and few patients survive more than 3 years after the disease is identified (Curran, Morgan, Starcher, Hardy, & Jaffe, 1985).

1.2.2. AIDS-Related Complex

As noted earlier, AIDS is defined by the presence of clear-cut disease predictive of defective cell-mediated immunity in the absence of a known cause for diminished resistance to that disease. Kaposi's sarcoma, pneumocystic *carinii* pneumonia, and many of the diseases just described meet this surveillance criterion. However, far more HIV-infected persons show symptoms of illness related to immune system compromise than show full evidence of AIDS that meets the CDC surveillance definition. Establishing the proper medical/diagnostic classification for these individuals has proven difficult from the beginning of the health epidemic. Initially, persons with HIV infection accompanied by symptoms of immunosuppression, but falling short of clear-cut AIDS, were considered to have *Pre-AIDS, Prodromal AIDS,* or *Lesser AIDS* diseases. These terms have generally been discarded, in part because the assumption that all immunocompromised persons invariably develop full-blown AIDS is

TABLE 2
Classifications of HIV Infections

Group I Acute infection	Mononucleosislike syndrome associated with recent HIV infection
Group II Asymptomatic infection	HIV infection but no clinical signs or symptoms

Group III
  Persistent generalized
  lymphadenopathy
	Lymph node enlargement (1 mm or more at two or more extrainguinal sites for more than 3 months without cause other than HIV infection)

Group IV	
Subgroup A	Constitutional disease (persistent fever, wasting,, diarrhea) due to HIV infection
Subgroup B	Neurological disease (dementia, neuropathy, myelopathy) due to HIV infection
Subgroup C	Infectious diseases secondary to HIV infection (viral, fungal, bacterial, parasitic), including pneumocystic pneumonia
Subgroup D	Cancers secondary to HIV infection, including Kaposi's sarcoma, lymphoma, and others
Subgroup E	Other diseases secondary to HIV infection

questionable. The term *AIDS-related complex* (ARC) has been frequently used to designate diseases and clinical symptoms of immunosuppression without the massive opportunistic illnesses characteristic of AIDS. ARC is a descriptor still widely used in the literature, but it is of limited precision because it encompasses so many different symptoms and illnesses with varying degrees of severity and varying prognoses.

The Centers for Disease Control proposed a classification system for HIV infections that is likely to be increasingly adopted by clinicians and researchers (*Centers for Disease Control*, 1986b). Table 2 summarizes this system, which creates four major groups based on infection status. Group I (acute infection) includes persons with transient symptoms associated with initial HIV infection. Group II (asymptomatic infection) refers to persons who are HIV-infected but show no signs or symptoms of clinical illness. Group III is reserved for patients with persistent generalized lymphadenopathy but not other clinical symptoms. Group IV, a more complicated classification for patients with HIV-related diseases, is divided into five subcategories based on the type of disease (constitutional disease; neurological disease; secondary infections of a viral, bacterial, parasitic, or fungal nature; secondary cancers; and other conditions related to HIV infection). AIDS is always represented by a Group IV diagnosis, while patients with ARC are classified into either Group III (if they have only persistent generalized lymphadenopathy) or, potentially, one of the Group IV categories. This system is useful because it provides a means to categorize HIV diseases more precisely than is possible with an AIDS/ARC distinction alone. Moreover, it refocuses attention that the critical aspects of the AIDS health crisis are HIV infection and the wide range of illnesses with different clinical expressions that are related to HIV infection.

1.3. INCIDENCE AND DEMOGRAPHY

From the time when AIDS was first identified, two aspects of the syndrome were clear: AIDS cases have increased at a rapid and, at times, exponential rate, and AIDS is much more likely to affect persons in specific risk categories than the population as a whole. In this section, we will first consider prevalence of the disease and then discuss risk groups most affected by it.

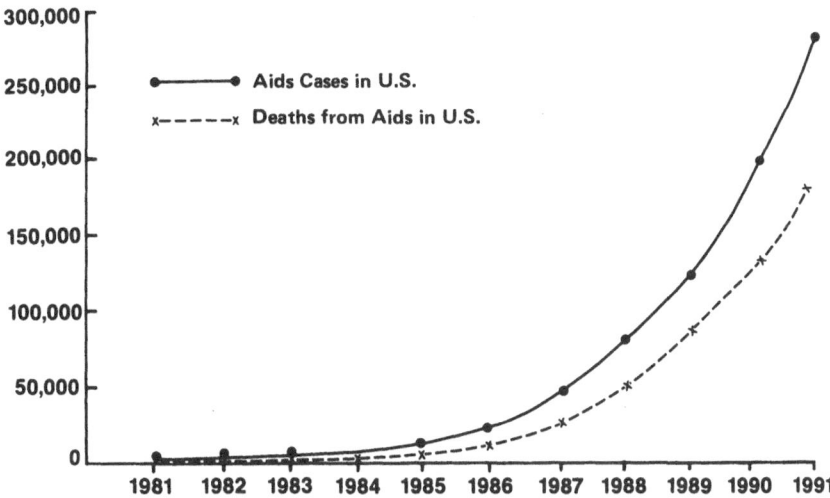

FIGURE 1. Past and projected number of AIDS cases and AIDS deaths in the United States, 1981–1991. (*Source:* U.S. Department of Health and Human Services.)

1.3.1. AIDS Incidence and Prevalence

From 1979 to 1980, 62 persons in the United States were identified as victims of what would shortly be called AIDS. In 1981, 239 AIDS cases were diagnosed; in 1982, 961 were diagnosed; and in 1983, 2,501 new cases of AIDS were identified. The prevalence of AIDS has continued to escalate steadily and rapidly since those years. By mid-1987, the number of AIDS cases in the United Stated reported to the CDC was approximately 50,000 (Centers for Disease Control, 1987). Approximately 10 times the number of AIDS patients, or about 500,000 Americans, exhibit clinical symptoms of immune system impairment or ARC (Fauci, 1986). Recent projections that take into account past incidence of the disease and current prevalence of HIV infection indicate that by 1991, 270,000 cases of full-blown AIDS will have been diagnosed in the United States (U.S. Department of Health and Human Services, 1986a). If this projection proves accurate, acquired immune deficiency syndrome will soon rank as one of the country's leading causes of death for males under age 40. If the number of persons becoming HIV-infected continues to increase and if a large percentage of those people HIV-infected eventually become ill, fatalities may ultimately reach staggering proportions (Figure 1).

The impact of AIDS is greatest on persons who are relatively young, since approximately 70% of AIDS victims are under 39 years of age. Sixty percent of adult AIDS patients are white, 25% black, and 14% Hispanic, reflecting a disproportionate prevalence of the syndrome among minorities. Ninety-three percent of current AIDS patients in the United States are males (Centers for Disease Control, 1987).

When AIDS first appeared, it was largely confined to large cities such as New York, Newark, Houston, San Francisco, Los Angeles, and Miami. These geographical areas continue to have the greatest number of cases. However, AIDS appears regularly in all states, and prevalence of the disease has increased dramatically in every part of the country. The notion that a few large cities are "dangerous" with respect to AIDS but that smaller cities are "safe" may have been true at the very start of the epidemic. However, the number of HIV-infected persons has greatly increased in all areas. AIDS has also now been diagnosed in most countries in the world, although imprecision in case-monitoring mechanisms and underreporting in some nations for political, social, and economic reasons make it difficult to obtain accurate worldwide prevalence data. However, it is clear that many millions of persons across different areas of the world are already infected.

1.3.2. Risk Groups

Approximately 95% of present American AIDS patients fall within one of five identified risk groups. The largest risk group, which accounts for 65% of all adult AIDS cases, is homosexual or bisexual men. Gay men who are also intravenous drug users account for approximately 8% of additional AIDS cases, while heterosexual intravenous drug users represent approximately 17% of AIDS cases. Hemophiliacs (1%), other persons with a history of blood transfusions (2%), and individuals who contracted AIDS during heterosexual activities (4%) represent other high-risk groups (Centers for Disease Control, 1986c). The approximately 3% of American AIDS cases that do not fall within one of these groups may include persons who are not candid concerning their risk experiences and persons sexually exposed to AIDS without their awareness.

Several issues concerning AIDS risk categories merit comment. First, AIDS risk groups are not static. Early in the epidemic, Haitians were considered to be a risk group; later epidemiological studies showed the designation of Haitians as a separate AIDS risk category to be unjustified.

The large majority of AIDS cases are homosexual and bisexual males, and this pattern is likely to continue. The already small percentage of hemophiliac and blood transfusion-related cases of AIDS should eventually decline following the institution several years ago of blood bank HIV-antibody screening. On the other hand, heterosexual cases of AIDS are expected to increase as a result of transmission during heterosexual activities. As the number of heterosexual female AIDS cases increases, pediatric cases may also increase owing to viral transmission to the fetus by pregnant HIV-infected women. Changes in demographics will probably be detected gradually since the latency from HIV exposure to clinical disease onset is long, and they will be preceded by changes in HIV-antibody positivity rates for the affected populations. The implementation of wide-scale prevention and behavior change programs could serve to alter AIDS risk group demographics, as we will discuss in detail later.

It should also be noted that all members of groups at risk for AIDS do not share the same level of AIDS exposure risk. Homosexual or bisexual males who do not engage in sexual activities that permit HIV transmission are not, theoretically, at any greater exposure risk than members of the general population. Gay males who are celibate, those who maintain an exclusive sexual relationship with a partner who is not HIV-exposed, and those who diligently adopt sexual practices that do not permit efficient HIV transfer are not at high risk for sexually transmitted HIV exposure (Detels, Visscher, Kingsley, & Chmiel, 1987; Jaffe, Hardy, Morgan, & Darrow, 1985; Kingsley et al., 1987). In similar fashion, intravenous drug users are at risk for AIDS exposure only when they share or reuse needles and are therefore exposed to HIV-infected blood from previous users of the same needle. Thus, AIDS transmission occurs as a function of the exposure risk behavior of people rather than because of membership in a high-risk group. We will pursue the implications of this for AIDS prevention over the next several chapters.

AIDS has proven to be not only a lethal but an unusual disease, remaining much more highly contained within identifiable risk groups than most other viral infections owing to its narrow avenues of transmission. This is fortunate since it means that many persons are unlikely to be exposed to HIV or contract AIDS. However, for individuals within both past and future AIDS risk groups, the effects of the disease are devastating. The persons most likely to be the victims of AIDS, gay males, were negatively stigmatized even before the AIDS epidemic, and homophobic prejudice, combined with the belief that AIDS is unlikely to affect most heterosexuals, no doubt lessened the vigor of constructive early response to the health crisis. Whether AIDS risk categories remain relatively constant or whether they eventually expand to include additional groups of people, it is increasingly clear that acquired immune deficiency syndrome is the most serious infectious disease epidemic of modern times.

Transmission and Risk Factors for AIDS

As we discussed in Chapter 1, HIV transmission occurs when the virus from an infected individual's body fluids, primarily blood or semen, gains entry to the bloodstream of another person. Among some AIDS risk groups, the reasons for increased HIV susceptibility are readily apparent. Hemophiliacs and transfusion recipients were directly exposed to the virus if they received blood or blood products contaminated with HIV. The likelihood of developing HIV infection if one received contaminated blood is high in light of follow-up studies of transfusion recipients (Ward *et al.*, 1987), although the likelihood that a transfusion recipient received contaminated blood even before antibody screening was instituted is quite low. Intravenous drug users who share needles inject themselves with blood traces from persons who previously used the same syringe. If a previous user of the needle carried the virus, HIV transmission can occur. In a similar manner, HIV-infected females who become pregnant can give birth to infants infected with the virus because the blood-borne virus circulates between the mother and the fetus (Oleske *et al.*, 1983; Rubenstein *et al.*, 1983). Virtually all pediatric AIDS cases occur either because the child was exposed prenatally to the virus via its mother's bloodstream, because the child was exposed during delivery, or because the child received transfusions of infected blood (U.S.

Department of Health and Human Services, 1986a). However, as we noted in the previous chapter, transfusion with contaminated blood accounts for only a small proportion of the total number of AIDS cases. The vast majority of AIDS patients and of persons antibody-positive to the virus were exposed as a result of sexual transmission.

2.1. AIDS RISK BEHAVIOR AMONG HOMOSEXUAL OR BISEXUAL MALES

Most early studies of AIDS risk behavior among gay and bisexual males employed retrospective methodologies, questioning persons within established clinical groups (AIDS, ARC, or HIV seropositivity) about their past sexual or health practices and then comparing their responses with those of healthy or HIV-seronegative control groups. This methodology was useful for initially identifying behavioral correlates of AIDS and HIV infection. However, retrospective studies are limited by their reliance on self-reports of past behavior, by potential ambiguities in the definition of behavior or the recall of subjects, by confounds caused if control and experimental groups are not fully matched on all relevant variables, and by the inability to definitively establish causal relationships between subjects' past behavior and their current health status. More recent prospective studies of AIDS risk have now been conducted and, when considered together with the findings of laboratory investigations, elucidate major transmissions mechanisms. The risk factors most frequently identified among homosexual or bisexual males are number of sexual partners, specific sexual practices engaged in with sexual partners, history of certain sexually transmitted diseases, and substance use history.

2.1.1. Number of Sexual Partners

If HIV infection is present in some proportion of the sexually active gay male population and if the virus can be sexually transmitted, the likelihood of an individual's exposure to HIV should vary with the number of sex partners encountered. Several investigations have demonstrated such an effect. Marmor *et al.* (1982) found that patients with AIDS had significantly more different sexual partners during the year before their disease was diagnosed than did age- and race-matched homosexual male controls without AIDS. Similar results were obtained in a larger-scale study by Groopman, Mayer, *et al.* (1985). In addition to these retrospective studies, Anderson and Levy (1985) conducted a prospective investigation and found that frequency of sexual partners over a 2-year period significantly predicted HIV seropositivity. Taken together, these studies suggest that individuals who have more sexual partners may stand a greater likelihood of encountering the virus.

However, not all investigations have found an independent association between number of different sexual partners and AIDS or HIV seropositivity (Calabrese *et al.*, 1985; Detels *et al.*, 1983). There are several possible reasons why number of different sex partners may no longer be a consistent, independent AIDS risk predictor. When the prevalence of HIV infection among sexually active gay males was quite low, contact with many different partners would be needed for an individual to encounter an infected partner. Early in the health epidemic, anecdotal reports indicated that some AIDS patients had hundreds of different sexual partners prior to the onset of their illness (Jaffe, Bregman, & Selik, 1985). However, the prevalence of HIV infection has greatly increased among the sexually active gay male population in most areas (Anderson & Levy, 1985; Carlson *et al.*, 1985; Lang *et al.*, 1987) and few sex partner contacts are now needed to encounter an HIV-infected individual. A recent large-scale prospective study of gay or bisexual men found that HIV seroconversion from antibody-negative to antibody-positive status required very few occurrences of high-risk conduct with different partners (Kingsley *et al.*, 1987). Men who had five or more high-risk contacts in a 1-year period were 18 times more likely to become HIV-infected than those men who did not engage in high-risk practices with multiple partners. Thus, promiscuity or sheer number of different partners is now a relatively less salient independent risk predictor for gay or bisexual men than it was early in the AIDS crisis.

2.1.2. High-Risk Sexual Practices

Since HIV transmission requires that the virus from an infected individual's blood or semen enter the partner's bloodstream, sexual practices that permit bloodstream access presumably carry higher HIV infection risk than practices that do not permit efficient bloodstream entry. A number of sexual activities have emerged as AIDS risk predictors.

2.1.2.1. Unprotected Anal Intercourse

Across numerous studies, anal intercourse, and especially receptive anal intercourse, has been identified as the strongest predictor of AIDS and HIV infection (Blattner, Biggar, Weiss, Melbye, & Goedert, 1985; Detels *et al.*, 1987; Goedert & Blattner, 1985; Groopman, Mayer, *et* al., 1985; Guinan, et al., 1984; Jaffe, Hardy, 1985; Kingsley et al., 1987; Melbye et al., 1984). From a physiological perspective, anal intercourse affords a high probability for HIV transmission because the rectal tears and trauma that often accompany this activity allow semen-borne virus to enter the bloodstream. Most studies show the receptive partner to be at a greater HIV exposure risk, although the insertive partner may also be exposed to the virus owing to contact with the partner's blood or body fluids.

In recent years, condom use has been widely advocated as a protection against HIV transmission during anal intercourse. Condoms have been shown to block passage of the virus in laboratory studies (Conant, Hardy, Sernatinger, Spicer, & Levy, 1986). Particularly when used in conjunction with spermicides or lubricants containing nonoxynol-9, a substance that inactivates HIV during in vitro tests, condoms appear to decrease significantly the likelihood of viral transmission during intercourse (Rietmeijer, Krebs, Feorino, & Judson, 1987; Scesney, Gantz, & Sullivan, 1987). However, the degree of protection afforded by condoms depends upon consistent, correct use and requires that the condom remain intact, unbroken, and undamaged during intercourse. Because condoms do occasionally fail or are used carelessly, and because anal intercourse is such a high-risk behavior, condom use probably affords a reasonable, but not necessarily an absolute, protection against HIV transmission during this activity (Kelly & St. Lawrence, 1987a).

2.1.2.2. Oral–Anal and Digital–Anal Contact

Both oral–anal ("rimming") and hand insertion in the rectum ("fisting") activities carry high HIV exposure risk, apparently for both the insertive and receptive partners (Goedert & Blattner, 1985; Jaffe, Darrow, et al., 1985; Newell et al., 1985). In addition, practices that involve sharing inserted rectal sex devices or any practices that permit bloodstream contact with partner's blood or body excretions should be considered high in risk for HIV transmission.

2.1.2.3. Oral–Genital Intercourse

Most epidemiological studies have failed to find a strong, consistent association between oral–genital activities and AIDS or HIV-positive status (Goedert & Blattner, 1985; Jaffe, Bregman, & Selik, 1985; Kingsley et al., 1987; Lyman, Ascher, & Levy, 1986; Newell et al., 1985); in general, receptive anal intercourse has been a much stronger risk predictor than receptive oral intercourse. However, there are several reasons to believe that oral–genital contact, especially to orgasm, may also present risk. First, the studies that have failed to establish this activity as an AIDS risk predictor have generally employed small samples or have examined subjects whose past sexual behavior included such a wide range of intertwined sexual activities that teasing out the independent definitive risk contribution of each activity is difficult. Second, oral–genital contact to orgasm would seem to afford the virus access to the bloodstream, especially if the recipient partner had oral cuts, abrasions, cold sores, periodontal disease, or other blood entry routes. Thus, while oral–genital contact has not emerged in epidemiology studies as a definitive risk factor, the activity should be considered a probable means of HIV transmission, especially if practiced to orgasm.

2.1.2.4. Deep Kissing

Following a report that HIV antibodies had been detected in saliva (Ho et al., 1985), concerns were raised that the virus might be transmissible through saliva exchange during "deep" kissing activities. No epidemiological studies have ever definitively implicated deep kissing as a primary activity responsible for HIV infection, perhaps because the virus is rarely present in saliva and, even when present, has been detected only at very low titres (Ho et al., 1985). In addition, social (dry") kissing clearly does not pose transmission risk (Friedland et al., 1986). Relative to the very high risk that is posed by such activities as unprotected intercourse, deep kissing does not appear to be a strong AIDS risk factor, although prudence concerning the activity has been encouraged (Fox & Baum, 1986; Voeller, 1986).

Just as there are many variations in heterosexual practices, there is diversity in the sexual activities that can occur between male partners. Attempting to catalog all possible homosexual activities and establish the specific level of HIV transmission risk associated with each represents a formidable task; it is unlikely that either epidemiological or laboratory studies will be able to fully explicate all sexual risk behaviors. In general, however, activities that permit blood, semen, or body fluid exchange are also high in transmission risk. The level of risk appears to vary depending on the likelihood that fluid-borne HIV can enter a partner's bloodstream. Sexual activities that carry lower exposure risk are those that do

TABLE 3

Probable Degree of HIV Transmission Risk Associated with Sexual Activities among Gay or Bisexual Males

High risk	Probable moderate risk	Probable low risk[a]	No risk
Anal intercourse without condom	Anal intercourse with condom (risk due to breakage potential)	Mutual masturbation	Celibacy
Oral–anal activity	Oral–genital activity	Massage	Maintenance of sexually exclusive relationship when neither partner is HIV-exposed
Digital-anal ("fisting") activity		Rubbing or friction activities (frottage) without insertion	
Other practice that could entail bloodstream exposure to partner's excretions, or semen			

[a]Each of the above is lowest in risk when partners do not come in contact with the semen, blood, or other body fluids of partner

not entail fluid exchange or permit ready bloodstream entry to the virus. Such "safer sex" activities between male partners include condom use, mutual masturbation, massage, rubbing or friction ("frottage") contact without insertion, and similar practices. Preliminary empirical research (Detels *et al.*, 1987) now suggests that gay or bisexual individuals who refrain from high-risk activities and consistently adopt these safer sex practices are at reduced risk for HIV infection. However, even safer sex practices may present exposure risk under some circumstances. Although HIV does not penetrate intact skin, cuts or abrasions on skin surfaces could afford a potential entry route for the virus even during noninsertive sex between partners. The most appropriate way to conceptualize the HIV transmission risk of homosexual activities is along a continuum ranging from those practices likely to allow virus transmission if one partner is infected to those practices that are unlikely to permit virus transfer even if one partner is HIV-infected (Table 3).

2.1.3. History of Sexually Transmitted Diseases

A number of studies have found that history of sexually transmitted diseases is a risk factor for AIDS (Guinan *et al.*, 1984; Jaffe *et al.*, 1983; Kingsley *et al.*, 1987; Marmor *et al.*, 1982; Newell *et al.*, 1985; Weber *et al.*, 1986. The sexually transmitted diseases identified as AIDS risk predictors include prior syphilis, gonorrhea, mononucleosis, cytomegalovirus, hepatitis, and certain intestinal parasitic diseases. Some investigators have theorized that the development of AIDS is more likely to occur in persons with a prior history of sexually transmitted diseases owing to interactional or potentiating effects of HIV with those other infections (Sonnabend *et al.*, 1985). However, an alternative explanation is that individuals who engage in high-risk sexual activities with multiple partners are likely to be exposed not only to "traditional" sexually transmitted diseases but also to HIV. This is especially plausible since the sexual activities that can result in transmission of gonorrhea, syphilis, and hepatitis are generally the same activities that permit the efficient transmission of HIV.

2.1.4. Substance Use History

Apart from HIV transmission among intravenous drug users who share needles, research attention has focused on the role of chemical substance use as a risk factor for AIDS. Among the substances that have been identified as differentially associated with AIDS are cigarette smoking, marijuana smoking, and the use of inhaled nitrites (Marmor *et al.*, 1982; Newell *et al.*, 1985; Weber *et al.*, 1986). Of these substances, the greatest attention has focused on the possible role of inhaled nitrites as an AIDS risk cofactor (Goedert, 1985; Newell *et al.*, 1985).

Amyl, butyl, and isobutyl nitrites ("poppers") are vasodilators that produce transient hypotension, flushing, light-headedness, and anesthesia when inhaled. Amyl nitrites have long been used therapeutically to provide relief from angina pectoris, but in the 1970s they became available in nonprescription form and were used by some persons in the homosexual community for sexual pleasure enhancement. There is evidence, based largely on animal studies, that inhaled nitrites are carcinogenic, and there are limited corelational data suggesting that nitrite use may be associated with T-lymphocyte abnormalities in humans (Dax, Adler, Nagel, Dorsey, & Jaffe, 1987; Goedert, 1985; Newell *et al.*, 1985). For these reasons, and because the use of inhaled nitrites as a recreational drug substantially increased in the gay community just prior to the AIDS epidemic, some investigators suspect that nitrites may play a role in the development of AIDS. However, this linkage is speculative and is based largely on correlational data; lesbians who use nitrites heavily are not at risk for AIDS, and increased AIDS risk has not been reported among angina patients who use nitrite inhalants therapeutically.

The physiological risk-potentiating effects from nitrite inhalation cannot be ruled out and merit further evaluation. However, their role in AIDS etiology may be behavioral rather than chemical. Inhaled nitrite use is especially common among individuals who engage in such high-risk sexual activities as receptive anal intercourse, perhaps because of its behavior-disinhibiting and mildly anesthetic effects (Siegel, Mesagno, Chen, & Christ, 1987; Stall, McKusick, Wiley, Coates, & Ostrow, 1986; Stevens, Taylor, Rodriguez, & Rubenstein, 1987). Thus, an association between AIDS and inhaled nitrites may be due primarily to the correlation of drug use with high-risk sexual activities. Further, amyl, butyl and isobutyl nitrites are potent vasodilators. If an individual engages in a sexual activity that involves fluid exchange while using nitrites, increased blood flow and vasodilation following nitrite inhalation could well afford an increased opportunity for HIV entry.

Excessive alcohol consumption and the use of marijuana and other drugs at the time of sexual activity are also related to increased probability of engaging in high-risk sexual practices. In a large-scale prospective investigation, Stall *et al.* (1986) found that gay men in San Francisco who adhered to "safer sex" practice recommendations were less likely to use chemical substances during or immediately preceding sexual activities. Risk-reduction behavior changes made by subjects over a 1-year period were also significantly correlated with a reduction in the use of intoxicants and drugs during sex. Thus, although the chronic, heavy use of alcohol and other drugs itself can produce immune system impairment (Lundy *et al.*, 1975; Young, Van der Weyden, Rose, & Dudley, 1979), it appears more likely that substance use contributes to risk through disinhibition, the induction of poor judgment, or other behavioral processes for susceptible persons (Stall *et al.*, 1986; Stevens *et al.*, 1987).

Whether chemical substances such as inhaled nitrites, excessive alcohol or marijuana intake, or the use of other recreational drugs might play some causative role in the development of AIDS or its opportunistic infections is not known at present. However, to the degree that these substances produce sexual disinhibition and impaired judgment, their use or overuse can clearly influence the likelihood that an individual will engage in sexual activities that might result in HIV exposure or transmission.

2.2. AIDS RISK BEHAVIOR AMONG HETEROSEXUALS

As we saw in Chapter 1, approximately 25% of American AIDS patients are heterosexual. Of these, the large majority fall into risk categories described earlier (intravenous drug users, hemophiliacs, and blood transfusion recipients). However, approximately 5% of current AIDS patients are heterosexuals who do not apparently belong to identifiable risk groups (Centers for Disease Control, 1987). Presumably, most of these are individuals exposed to HIV as a result of heterosexual contact.

In the areas of central Africa where HIV infection is highly prevalent, the majority of persons exposed to the virus and who develop AIDS are heterosexual and do not have a history of blood transfusions, homosexual activity, or drug use (Clumeck *et al.*, 1984, 1985; Van de Perre *et al.*, 1984). In contrast to current AIDS epidemiology in Western countries, females appear to be affected by the disease to an extent equal to that of males (Piot *et al.*, 1984). While comprehensive, large-scale risk factor studies on AIDS among central Africans have not yet been conducted, preliminary investigations to date revealed the association of AIDS, generalized lymphadenopathy, and HIV-exposed status with heterosexual promiscuity (Clumeck *et al.*, 1985; Katzenstein, Latif, Bassett, & Emmanuel, 1987; Plummer *et al.*, 1987; Van de Perre *et al.*, 1984). In these studies, a history of vaginal intercourse with multiple partners most frequently distinguishes HIV-infected and noninfected persons. Although it is possible that the reuse of contaminated needles in some inoculation campaigns or public health facilities in impoverished areas is responsible for occasional cases of AIDS, African surveillance data clearly implicate transmission of the virus through heterosexual activities.

Numerous case studies and several group investigations conducted in Western countries have also now established that HIV transmission occurs between heterosexual partners (Calabrese & Gopalakrishna, 1986; Fischl *et al.*, 1987; Groopman, Sarngadharan *et al.*, 1985; *Journal of the American Medical Association*, 1987a, 1987b; Redfield *et al.*, 1987; Wallace *et al.*, 1983). In countries where HIV infection is not yet prevalent in the general heterosexual population, the virus is most apt to affect heterosexual persons whose sexual partners are members of AIDS risk groups, such as bisexual males, intravenous drug users, or prostitutes. However, as the prevalence of HIV infection increases in the heterosexual population, linkages requiring direct sexual contact with persons in identified, "traditional" AIDS risk groups become less salient. Heterosexual persons who have had no personal sexual contact with risk group members, but whose sexual partners did, can become infected and can transmit the virus to others.

Definitive studies establishing the prevalence of HIV infection within the heterosexually active populations in the United States and other Western countries have not yet been undertaken. However, studies of HIV-seropositivity rates among blood donors (Schorr, Berkowitz, Cumming, Katz, & Sandler, 1985) and military personnel (Brundage *et al.*, 1987) indicate that fewer than 1% of persons in such mainstream populations are currently exposed to the virus. However, these data are not necessarily as reassuring as they appear. The actual prevalence of HIV infection among heterosexuals and the likelihood of heterosexual HIV transmission may depend on more fine-grained population characteristics. Heterosexuals in large cities are more likely to encounter partners who are, or who had previous sexual contact with, intravenous drug users because IV drug users tend to be concentrated in urban areas. Owing to geographical proximity with drug users, the urban poor may be at increased risk for heterosexual exposure to the virus. Unexpectedly high rates of HIV seropositivity have been reported in some isolated communities apparently owing to the combination of high rates of intravenous drug use and heterosexual promiscuity (Castro, Lieb, Galisher, Witte, & Jaffe, 1987).

There have now been several investigations of sexual behavior risk factors for AIDS and HIV infection among heterosexuals. Redfield *et al.* (1987) studied 15 male and female patients who acquired HIV diseases through contact with persons of the opposite sex. In some cases, subjects reported past sexual contact with opposite-sex persons who were intravenous drug users or who developed AIDS-related illnesses. However, the majority of persons in the Redfield *et al.* (1987) study simply reported large numbers of different heterosexual partners over the preceding 5-year period. The predominant sexual activity linked to HIV exposure was unprotected vaginal intercourse.

Fischl *et al.* (1987) also studied heterosexual transmission of HIV but did so by examining the antibody status of spouses of persons with AIDS. To be included in the study, the spouses without AIDS could themselves have no independent risk factors for the illness other than heterosexual contact with their partner. Fischl *et al.* (1987) found that 29% of spousal partners of persons with AIDS were antibody-positive to HIV when they entered the study. Fifty-eight percent became antibody-positive within 1 to 3 years. Evidence showed that both male-to-female and female-to-male transmission occurred in approximately equal proportions. The two activities most strongly associated with subsequent seroconversion of a previously unexposed spouse were vaginal and oral intercourse, and vaginal intercourse alone was sufficient to transmit the infection. Upon entry to the study, some couples abstained from intercourse and others had intercourse only when condoms were used. In no cases did previously antibody-negative spouses in the abstinent couples later develop HIV antibodies, and seroconversion occurred in only 1 of 10 couples where condoms were reportedly used during intercourse (Fischl *et al.*, 1987). Interestingly, and affirming that unprotected heterosexual intercourse was the sole vehicle for transmission, the investigators found that other members of the same households who were antibody-negative at the start of the study and were not sexual partners of the AIDS patient never became exposed to the virus.

This discovery, taken together with the results of other studies of heterosexual transmission (Calabrese & Gopalakrishna, 1986; Groopman,

Sarngadharan, *et al.*, 1985; Harris *et al.*, 1983; *Journal of the American Medical Association*, 1987a, 1987b; Wallace *et al.*, 1983), makes it evident that HIV infection can be transmitted both from males to females and from females to males during unprotected vaginal intercourse and, perhaps, during oral intercourse. Whether male-to-female transmission is more probably than female-to-male transmission is not clear.

It is difficult to draw inferences about the long-term course of a health epidemic when only short-term epidemiological findings exist. It is even more difficult to project how a disease like AIDS, when sexually transmitted, will ultimately affect the heterosexual population. However, if heterosexual transmission of the HIV virus occurs with even some of the efficiency that characterizes its transmission during certain homosexual activities, major risk-reduction efforts for heterosexual persons will also prove critical. Assuming that the number of heterosexual carriers is still relatively low, and the base rate prevalence of HIV infection among primarily heterosexual persons is therefore also relatively low, promiscuity is likely to be an initial exposure and risk predictor for heterosexuals just as it had been for homosexuals. We would predict, as well, that cases of heterosexually transmitted AIDS will initially be concentrated in larger cities where persons have the greatest probability of encountering an HIV-infected partner, and that increases in AIDS cases attributable to heterosexual transmission will be preceded by an increased prevalence of HIV seropositivity among this population. From such a perspective, the risk predictors of heterosexually transmitted AIDS would parallel the risk behaviors identified for homosexuals: frequent sexual encounters with different partners, engaging in activities that permit semen, blood, and body fluid exchange, and history of previous sexually transmitted diseases.

2.3. REDUCED-RISK CONDUCT

Because HIV transmission high-risk activities have been identified, low-risk alternative behaviors are also implied, and it is now possible to counsel individuals to reduce their exposure risk. As suggested earlier, risk levels are relative rather than absolute for risk group members who are sexually active. However, in addition to celibacy, homosexual or heterosexual persons are at no risk for HIV sexual transmission if they maintain an exclusive, monogamous relationship with one other person and if both partners are unexposed to the HIV virus. Unfortunately, these conditions may be difficult to ensure. Individuals can carry the HIV virus but test negative for HIV antibodies if an insufficient period of time has passed for antibodies to develop (Copper *et al.*, 1985). The issue of monogamy may also be problematic. Even in committed relationships, sexual activities outside the relationship can occur. If extrarelationship sexual activities do take place, an assumption of HIV exposure "safety" during sexual activities within the primary relationship is unwarranted.

Given the increased prevalence of HIV infection among sexually active homosexual males in all areas of the country, the single most critical behavior change to reduce AIDS risk is consistent adoption of sexual activities that are unlikely to permit HIV transmission regardless of the infection status of either partner. As shown in Table 3, sexual activities with no body fluid exchange or potential bloodstream contact reduce transmission risk. Penetrative activities using condoms also afford exposure protection if condoms are used properly and if they remain intact. Adoption of these "safer sex" activities represents an important way for gay males who remain sexually active to reduce HIV infection risk. The adoption of similar practices to reduce risk, including condom use during vaginal intercourse, is equally relevant for nonmonogamous heterosexuals or for heterosexuals with partners who may be HIV-exposed.

A reduced-risk life-style includes a reduction in the number of different sexual partners. As we discussed earlier, multiple partner contacts were probably a more important independent risk predictor for homosexual males earlier in the health crisis than at present. Relatively few partners are now needed in most areas for gay men to encounter a partner who is HIV-infected, so sexual practices have become a more salient risk factor. However, persons who engage in casual sexual activities with multiple partners may more frequently encounter partners who are coercive or who pressure high-risk sexual behavior. One might surmise that individuals who frequently engage in casual sexual activities are also relatively less knowledgeable about risk behavior or are less concerned about health. For that reason, and because casual sexual contacts are not apt to be characterized by a high degree of concern for the partner's long-term well-being, limiting the number of different sexual partners represents another risk-reduction goal.

The nontherapeutic use of injectable drugs is maladaptive and dangerous for many reasons. Cessation of IV drug use, or, at the very least, cessation of needle sharing by drug users, is essential in the prevention of AIDS. Finally, reduced-risk life-styles may entail curtailing the use of chemical substances that produce sexual disinhibition, poor judgment, and susceptibility to coercions to engage in high-risk behaviors. To the extent that an individual is more likely to engage in risky activities when impaired or disinhibited by excessive consumption of alcohol, marijuana, inhaled nitrites, or other recreational drugs (Stall *et al.*, 1986), reduction in the use of these substances may also produce reduced-risk behavior for HIV transmission or exposure. Thus, the aims of AIDS prevention efforts are to (1) encourage the adoption of monogamous or exclusive relationships when possible, (2) promote the adoption of sexual practices that are low in HIV transmission risk by sexually active persons at risk for AIDS, (3) encourage individuals to adopt steady relationships characterized by low-risk sexual practices rather than casual, anonymous, or promiscuous high-risk sexual behavior, and (4) when warranted, curtail the overuse of chemical substances or intoxicants associated with disinhibition and with high-risk sexual conduct. In Chapters 3 and 4, intervention methods that can help persons make such behavior changes will be discussed.

2.3.1. Misconceptions Concerning Risk Practices

Many therapists, the general public, and people themselves at risk share certain misconceptions about AIDS risk practices and exposure prevention. From a public health perspective, one of the most important misconceptions is that patients with identified AIDS are primarily responsible for transmitting the HIV virus to others. As we discussed earlier, the number of persons with asymptomatic HIV infection vastly exceeds the number of patients with identifiable AIDS or HIV-related illness. Since transmission of the virus can occur during high-risk activities with any HIV-infected person, regardless of that individual's clinical health, the majority of transmission episodes occur between people who appear to be in good health. Further, because most HIV-infected individuals do not show visible manifestations of their viral carrier status, a person's healthful appearance provides no information concerning HIV infection.

For these reasons, the most appropriate prevention objective is to encourage and assist persons to refrain from engaging in high-risk practices with any partner who might carry the HIV virus. Homosexual or bisexual males should presume that any male sexual partner is potentially HIV-infected and capable of transmitting the virus during high-risk activities. Men with a history of homosexual activities should assume that they themselves could be HIV-exposed and capable of passing it to others. Finally, heterosexually active persons with multiple partners should also take precautions to prevent transmission risk. To the extent that a heterosexual individual is unfamiliar with his or her sexual partner's possible risk factor background, risk precautions are especially salient.

2.4. THE CASE AGAINST CASUAL TRANSMISSION

Few diseases have elicited such a degree of fear and, at times, hysteria as has AIDS. During the past several years, proposals have been advanced to incarcerate; quarantine; deny employment, insurance, and housing; and even tattoo persons with AIDS or persons antibody-positive to HIV. In cities with a high prevalence of AIDS, episodes of violence directed against homosexuals have increased greatly, apparently owing to the public's association of AIDS with gay life-styles (National Gay and Lesbian Task Force, 1987). AIDS patients have been denied medical care or have encountered negativity, fear, and avoidance even by health care providers (Burda & Powills, 1986; McAuliffe, Carey, Wells, Quick, & Dobbin, 1987). Although there is reason to believe that antigay prejudice is responsible for some of these reactions and proposals (Ottenberg, 1986; St. Lawrence, Husfeldt, Kelly, Hood, & Smith, in press), it is also evident that much of the public continues to fear that AIDS can be contracted through casual, nonintimate, and everyday social contact.

The case against casual transmission of HIV is substantial. Unlike the rhinoviruses responsible for colds or various influenza viruses that are airborne and highly contagious, HIV is present only in certain body fluids and requires bloodstream access for transmission. Although HIV antibodies have occasionally been isolated from saliva or tears (Ho *et al.*, 1985), they are present in these fluids rarely and at very low concentrations. No cases of HIV infection have ever been linked to exposure to body fluids other than blood, blood products, semen, and possibly vaginal fluids. The HIV virus is fragile, survives for variable but brief periods in open air, and can be killed with common household disinfectants such as bleach (Jain *et al.*, 1987). The fact that AIDS is highly confined to identifiable risk groups where its prevalence can consistently be explained by sexual activity, drug use, or blood transfusion history provides further evidence against casual transmission. If the virus could be transmitted casually, such clear risk groups would not exist. There is no evidence that HIV can be contracted by touching, social kissing, shaking hands, breathing the same air, working in the same office, being served food, or even sharing a household with an AIDS patient or an HIV-infected person provided that risk activities or blood contact do not occur* (Fischl *et al.*, 1987; Friedland *et al.*, 1986; Friedland, Saltzman *et al.*, 1987).

Two large-scale studies empirically disconfirm the notion that AIDS can be casually contracted. Friedland *et al.* (1986) studied 101 close but nonsexual household contacts of 41 patients with AIDS or AIDS-related complex diseases. The household contacts included children, siblings, parents, and other relatives of the patients, and none were themselves members of AIDS risk groups. To be included, household members must have resided with the patient for 3 months or longer, although the median duration of household contact exceeded 31 months. Many of the household members reported assisting the patient in bathing, dressing, and eating, and over 90% shared the same toilet, bath, and kitchen. Friedland et al. (1986) examined both the clinical health and the HIV antibody status of all household contacts and found that only one household member—a 5-year-old whose mother had AIDS—was confirmed to be HIV antibody-positive. There was considerable evidence that this child contracted HIV infection either prenatally or shortly after birth rather than as a result of household contact. Thus, even close, daily interactions with AIDS patients affords no risk of casually transmitted infection (Fischl et al., 1987; Friedland et al., 1986; Friedland, Saltzman, et al., 1987).

Another large-scale project investigated occupational risk exposure among health care workers who had direct blood contact with AIDS and ARC patients (McCray, 1986). Subjects in the study were 451 phlebotomists, nurses, physicians, and other health care workers who had accidentally punctured themselves with needles contaminated with blood from an AIDS patient, were splashed with blood or other body fluids in the eye or on an open cut, or had other direct exposure. Subjects were followed for an average of 15 months following the accidents and were repeatedly tested for HIV antibodies and signs of immunodeficiency. Of

---

* In order to prevent accidental blood exposure, household members of HIV–infected persons are routinely advised to avoid sharing razors or toothbrushes and to avoid direct contact with blood or excretions.

the 451 subjects, only 2 became seropositive at any time for HIV antibodies and 1 of these was at risk because her sexual partner was an HIV-infected male. Thus, even for health care workers who have puncture accidents with contaminated needlesticks, and who would therefore seem to be at great accidental infection risk, the likelihood of developing HIV infection is very small and is much lower than the risk of developing hepatitis B under similar exposure circumstances (McCray, 1986).*

In light of these findings, it is evident that mental health and social service caregivers who have professional contact with AIDS patients and HIV-infected persons are not at exposure risk. Large-scale studies of the antibody status of health care workers such as nurses or physicians who have direct physical contact with AIDS patients reveal either no incidence of HIV infection in the workers (Gerberding, J. L., personal communication, cited in Sande, 1986) or an antibody-positive incidence that is lower than one finds in the general population (Centers for Disease Control, 1985b). Taken together, all of these investigations confirm that the HIV virus is not transmissible during ordinary social contact with an infected individual; that even persons who have close daily contact in a shared workplace, office, or home with AIDS patients are not at exposure risk provided blood exchange or high-risk sexual activities do not occur; and that mental health and social service professionals who treat AIDS patients are not at exposure risk.

*While these findings suggest that the likelihood of HIV transmission to health care workers is very low, precaution guidelines for workers having physical contact with HIV patients' body fluids and specimens have been developed and should be followed (Centers for Disease Control, 1985b, 1986d).

Risk-Reduction Counseling for Individuals and Groups

Individuals are not at risk for AIDS because of *who* they are. Gay men do not become exposed to HIV infection because they are homosexual, but rather only if they engage in specific high-risk sexual activities or engaged in those activities in the past and acquired the virus. In the same sense, intravenous drug use is dangerous but not with respect to AIDS unless the drug user shares needles. Because AIDS has been so closely identified with risk groups, there is often a tendency to assume that risk-group membership confers likelihood of developing the illness. It does not. Rather, it is engaging in certain identifiable behaviors that places persons at risk for AIDS.

The reliance on risk-group conceptualizations, although useful in identifying the initial epidemiology of AIDS, has perhaps outlived its usefulness. On the one hand, persons within various risk groups (e.g., gay men, intravenous drug users, or prostitutes) may believe that, simply because they are members of those groups, developing AIDS is inevitable. On the other hand, persons who are not in these groups may incorrectly feel "protected" from AIDS by virtue of their heterosexuality, the absence of an intravenous drug use history, or other factors. In either case, attention becomes deflected from the key point that behavior, rather than personal identity characteristics, is responsible for determining level of risk.

There is at present, and no doubt for years to come there will be, considerable public policy debate concerning the focus of AIDS prevention efforts. Some persons stress that the only certain means of avoiding sexually transmitted HIV exposure is the maintenance of either celibacy or a completely monogamous relationship with one other person when both are HIV-unexposed. Proponents of this viewpoint suggest that programs to prevent the spread of AIDS should stress the values of chastity until marriage, the maintenance of a lifelong marital relationship with the same person, and strict monogamy. Others note that it is naive to assume that most people now or in the future will successfully adopt such life-styles, and that prevention efforts should teach individuals to minimize their likelihood of HIV exposure regardless of their sexual preference, relationship fidelity, and so on.

The authors believe that it is important to assist all people in protecting themselves and others from HIV infection to the greatest extent possible. It is certainly wrong to argue against chastity, marriage, and monogamy for persons who choose and are able to maintain such life-styles. On the other hand, and for a variety of reasons, many individuals do not maintain this style of life and relationships. We believe it is essential that AIDS prevention efforts are based on the world as it is rather than on the world as some individuals might ideally wish it could be. Thus, while celibacy and lifelong monogamy are relationship choices made by certain people in response to their values, morals, relationship success, or fear of AIDS, persons not celibate or monogamous are no less deserving of the greatest degree of protection possible from the disease. Furthermore, because it is not possible to predict in advance persons' future sexual relationships and other life-style behavior, prevention efforts must be wide-scale and must focus directly on those steps that can be taken to minimize the likelihood of HIV transmission if the individual is, or when the individual becomes, sexually active.

Preventing AIDS and the spread of HIV infection has as its primary goal helping individuals reduce or eliminate those behaviors that place them at risk for HIV exposure, at risk for repeated future reexposures to the virus, or at risk for transmitting the virus to others if they are already infected. In Chapter 2, the topic of high- and low-risk behaviors was discussed. In this chapter, we will consider how therapists can assist individual clients or groups of clients in making behavior changes that will lessen their likelihood of HIV exposure and transmission. Chapter 4 will consider prevention strategies with the same objectives but which can be implemented on larger-scale, community-wide levels.

3.1. FOR WHOM ARE INDIVIDUAL AND GROUP PREVENTION EFFORTS NEEDED?

At this point in the health crisis, and because HIV infection is prevalent among sexually active gay males, men who engage in any high-risk activities with same-sex partners are at imminent threat for HIV exposure. Nonmonogamous heterosexual males and females are also at risk if they engage in unprotected intercourse, with risk level increasing as a function of the individual's number of different sexual partners. Number of different partners is probably a more salient independent risk factor for heterosexual persons than for homosexual males at present because the base rate prevalence of HIV infection is still much lower in the heterosexual population than in the gay male population (Brundage *et al.*, 1987; Hessol *et al.*, 1987). Thus, it requires fewer sexual contacts for gay men to encounter an HIV-infected partner than for a sexually active heterosexual to encounter a partner with HIV infection. However, this pattern is based only upon global statistical likelihoods. In areas where intravenous drug use, prostitution, and multiple partner contacts are more common, heterosexual transmission is also more probable (Castro *et al.,* 1987).

Mental health and health care professionals who see individuals in the course of their everyday practice come in contact with many clients who are at risk for HIV exposure, although risk reduction is rarely the primary reason these clients seek assistance. Ten percent of the adult male population is primarily homosexual, and a much larger percentage of persons have had some homosexual experience (Gadpaille, 1985; Kinsey, Pomeroy, & Martin, 1948). This means that well over 10% of the males seen in a medical, psychology, social work, or other mental health practice are at potential risk for AIDS if they are engaging in high-risk practices. Adding to this the sizable number of heterosexuals—perhaps the majority of heterosexuals under age 40—with multiple partners and persons who may use intravenous drugs, it is apparent that an extraordinarily large number of persons are at risk for HIV infection even though they and their health care providers may not be aware of it.

It can be argued that health and mental health care professionals should routinely assess all adolescent or adult clients for HIV risk knowledge and behavior, and should then provide risk-behavior-change counseling if it is needed. Professionals who see clients likely to be at increased risk—such as gay or bisexual men, heterosexual men or women with multiple partners, persons with a history of any "traditional" sexually transmitted diseases, persons with significant drug use histories, or individuals suspected of increased risk for these reasons—have an obligation to offer risk-reduction counseling even if fear of AIDS is not the primary reason the client sought therapy or assistance. Discussion of AIDS risk reduction is likely to be more productive and comfortable if the professional first establishes rapport with the client or patient, maintains a nonjudgmental demeanor, provides information on practical risk-reduction steps, answers client questions openly and honestly, and is perceived as genuinely concerned about the client's well-being. Because discussion of AIDS risk behavior necessarily entails candid discussion about sexual practices, the professional should be careful to avoid embarrassing the client and must maintain the confidentiality of any information that is discussed or revealed. In many states, major AIDS risk behaviors not only are stigmatizing but also involve what are statutorily illegal activities. Failure to diligently keep client confidences is unethical and also highly damaging to AIDS-prevention efforts.

3.2. PROVIDING RISK-REDUCTION INFORMATION

In order for individuals to reduce their likelihood for HIV exposure or transmission, it is important that high-risk practices be fully understood, that lower-risk alternatives be identified clearly, and that misconceptions concerning risk be corrected. When the authors counsel persons concerning risk reduction, we stress that risk levels are relative rather than absolute and that the only complete assurances against sexually transmitted HIV infection are celibacy or monogamy when both partners are HIV-unexposed. For persons who are neither celibate nor in an assuredly monogamous relationship, we identify practices associated with varying levels of risk based on epidemiological research to date. Because of the serious consequences of HIV infection, it is prudent to be conservative when suggesting that practices are "low risk." High-risk practices have been well identified in the research literature, but empirical studies confirming the relative safety of low-risk practices are less common. In addition, we believe it is responsible to identify practices as high risk when they could be high in risk for *either* partner. For example, rather than suggest that the insertive partner in unprotected anal intercourse is at relatively lower risk than the receptive partner, we advise persons to refrain from engaging in unprotected anal intercourse altogether. This results in greater protection for both partners, rather than tacitly encouraging persons to behave in ways that might be relatively safe for them but highly dangerous for their sexual partners.

Given the high prevalence of HIV infection among sexually active gay men and the increasing prevalence of infection among sexually active heterosexuals, it is important that persons assume that their sexual partners could be HIV-exposed and behave in ways that minimize their own exposure risk if they choose to remain sexually active. It is equally important that the individual being counseled assume that he or she could also be HIV-exposed unless there are definitive antibody test results to the contrary. These assumptions are primarily intended not to create unnecessary anxiety but rather to encourage individuals to behave responsibly, taking steps to protect both themselves and any sexual partners.

3.2.1. Providing Risk-Reduction Information to Gay Male and At-Risk Heterosexual Clients

Although it might seem that homosexual or bisexual men and at-risk heterosexuals would require different kinds of risk-reduction information, this is not the case. With only a few exceptions, high-risk practices for both groups are quite similar. In addition, and as will be discussed in Chapter 9, persons who are primarily homosexual often engage in some heterosexual activities, while predominantly heterosexual persons sometimes engage in homosexual activities (Padian, Wiley, & Winkelstein, 1987). Consequently, prevention information should be of sufficient breadth to address the diversity of human sexual behavior.

3.2.1.1. Educating Clients Concerning AIDS

Providing basic information about HIV infection constitutes the first component of counseling to reduce AIDS risk. This can include information about the relationship of HIV infection to AIDS and other HIV illnesses, the latency between HIV exposure and onset of illness, asymptomatic HIV states, estimated prevalence of HIV infection, and body fluids in which the virus is most concentrated. When clients are being counseled after learning of a positive HIV-antibody test, they often have more specific questions about health course and experience more fears, anxieties, and emotional distress that also require counseling. Strategies for assisting HIV-positive persons are discussed in greater detail in Chapter 6.

3.2.1.2. Identification of High-Risk Practices

Rather than attempt to catalog every high-risk sexual practice in isolation, which can easily confuse clients, we find it useful to first explain more general rationales concerning risk. For example, clients might be told that because semen and blood are the major fluids in which HIV is carried, any activity that permits semen or blood from one partner to gain entry into the body or bloodstream of another is high in risk. "Avoiding the exchange of body fluids " is an example of another general risk-reduction rationale. From the general can follow an identification of more specific high-risk sexual practices. Unprotected anal, vaginal, or oral intercourse (e.g., engaging in these activities without the protection of a condom) are activities that we counsel all at-risk individuals to avoid, although oral–genital contact not to orgasm is lower in HIV risk than unprotected intercourse to climax (Coates *et al.*, 1987). Reasons why these activities are unsafe should also be explained, noting how blood-to-bloodstream or semen-to-bloodstream contact could occur in each of them (Siegel, Grodsky, & Herman, 1986). Other activities also high in transmission risk (oral–anal contact, "fisting," sharing of sexual stimulation objects, or practices that might result in bloodstream access to feces or urine) are probably less common but merit discussion with the individual being counseled.

3.2.1.3. Identification of Lower-Risk Practices

The use of condoms, preferably in conjunction with a spermicicle/ lubricant containing at least a 0.5 percent concentration of nonoxynol-9, is one of the most practical steps individuals can take in reducing the likelihood of HIV transmission or exposure (Rietmeijer *et al.*, 1987; Scesney *et al.*, 1987) Persons at risk for HIV infection who engage in penetrative activities should be counseled to do so only when protection is afforded by a condom. If the individual is not familiar with condoms, he should be advised to practice using them correctly before any sexual activity takes place in order to lessen the likelihood of condom failure due to incorrect use. Oil-based lubricants deteriorate and weaken latex, so only water-based products are appropriate with condoms.

Condoms greatly reduce the likelihood that HIV transmission can take place during intercourse relative to the probability of transmission during unprotected intercourse. However, it is important to counsel individuals that even condoms afford only a relative degree of protection (Kelly & St. Lawrence, 1987a). An extensive body of contraception research indicates that, among heterosexual couples who rely on condoms for birth control, pregnancy occurs from 1% to as much as 15% of the time over a 1 year period (Katchadourian & Lunde, 1972; Trussell, Bloom & Pebley, 1981). Presumably, this failure is attributable to condom breaks or leaks, slippage, and improper use. Because condoms are not fully reliable for contraception purposes, owing to the possibility of occasional failure, we believe that they should not be considered safe, in an absolute sense, with respect to AIDS prevention either. This caution is especially relevant for persons whose partners are likely to be HIV-infected and for sexual practices, such as anal intercourse, that are very high in risk if accidental condom failure should occur (Kelly & St. Lawrence, 1987a).

HIV transmission requires an efficient bloodstream entry route. Therefore, sexual activities that do not entail penetration are much lower in risk than penetrative practices. Mutual masturbation, massage, and frottage (body rubbing without insertion) do not usually afford a ready entry route for HIV provided that body fluids do not come in contact with open cuts or skin breaks. These nonpenetrative activities are presumed to be exceedingly low in risk when condoms are also used or when the partners do not otherwise have direct contact with one another's body fluids.

When counseling at-risk individuals, it is critical to stress the importance of consistently adopting "safer sex" practices at all times and with all partners. Especially for gay men, simply reducing somewhat the frequency of high-risk activities is an insufficient risk-reduction strategy because of the substantial possibility that a partner will be HIV-infected. This implies the need not only for a quantitative reduction in the number of different sexual partners but also for a qualitative change in the types of sexual activities that take place between partners. Recent research indicates that gay men in committed relationships are less likely to adhere to safer sex practices with their regular relationship partner than are men who have casual sexual contacts (McKusick, Coates, Wiley, Morin, & Stall, 1987). This is problematic since HIV transmission can occur be-

TABLE 4
Frequent Misconceptions about AIDS Risk Behavior

Misconception	Correction
AIDS exposure likelihood can be meaningfully reduced by asking a partner about his/her sexual or drug use background.	Persons are unlikely to be candid about all aspects of their past conduct. Even if a partner is not a risk group member, he/she may have unknowingly become HIV-exposed by a previous partner who was infected. Except in monogamous relationships, it is necessary to presume the seropositivity of oneself and one's partner.
A person's physical appearance provides evidence of his/her HIV status.	The vast majority of HIV carriers are asymptomatic, with no evidence of illness, but are nonetheless capable of transmitting HIV infection to others.
Receptive anal intercourse is the only sexual practice that should be avoided to lessen AIDS risk.	While unprotected anal intercourse is extremely high in risk, HIV transmission can occur during other penetrative activities as well.
When a monogamous relationship is established, reduced-risk sexual practices are no longer important.	If either partner has been sexually active in the past, he/she may already be HIV-exposed. The only time "safer sex" practices need not be followed are when both partners are known to be unexposed to HIV and when both partners remain completely monogamous.
One antibody test can conclusively establish HIV seronegativity.	Because it may require several months for an HIV-exposed person to develop sufficient antibodies to produce a reactive (positive) test, a single negative ELISA or Western blot finding suggests, but does not completely establish, seronegativity. Repeated testing, with no occurrence of risk activity between tests, is needed to fully establish seronegative HIV status.
Because an individual has engaged in frequent past high-risk conduct, exposure has probably already taken place and behavior change is less important.	A significant proportion of people, even those in high-risk groups, are not yet exposed to HIV. Even if an individual has been exposed, avoiding reexposure prevents the individual from repeated reinocculations of the virus; this may bear on health. Persons who may be HIV-exposed have a responsibility to protect the welfare of both themselves and their partners.
Showering before or after sexual activity is sufficient to reduce risk	Showering is prudent to remove any residue before or after sex. However, reduction in high-risk sexual practices is still critical.
Exercising, eating nutritiously, and getting enough rest can prevent AIDS	It is wise for all persons, especially those who are HIV-exposed or potentially exposed, to maintain good health and fitness. However, HIV can be transmitted even between persons in excellent fitness, so reduced-risk sexual practices must still be followed.

tween committed partners unless both are assuredly HIV-unexposed and remain monogamous. The adoption of lower-risk practices, even in the context of stable or committed sexual relationships, is clearly a prudent counseling goal for homosexual men in most circumstances. Finally, the therapist counseling a person who is at risk should be aware of misconceptions that a client may have concerning AIDS. Table 4 lists some of these common misconceptions and the reasons why they are inaccurate.

Because counseling individuals concerning risk reduction entails providing a great deal of information that might not be fully understood or recalled, the therapist may wish to provide supplementary written materials that emphasize the same points. Most health departments, public health service agencies, and AIDS clinics can supply informational brochures at no charge or at a nominal cost.

3.2.2. Providing Risk-Reduction Information to Clients Who Are Intravenous Drug Users

Although users of injected drugs such as heroin, cocaine, and amphetamines are found across all socioeconomic strata, intravenous drug use is most concentrated in the impoverished neighborhoods of large cities. Even in these areas, chronic intravenous drug users are often on the "outskirts" of mainstream community structures. As a result, IV drug users are an exceedingly difficult group to identify and target for either education or counseling efforts.

In the case of persons at risk for HIV infection as a result of high-risk sexual activities, only sexual practices must be changed in order to reduce the individual's likelihood of HIV exposure or transmission. However, for intravenous drug users, two risk factors are salient: transmission that results from needle sharing, and, once they are infected, creation of risk for their sexual partners. Individuals addicted to intravenous drugs are likely to be less responsive to health messages and counseling than most groups and may constitute a primary "bridge" for sexual HIV transmission to the heterosexual population. Theoretically, intravenous drug users can avoid HIV infection risk by refraining from needle sharing with others. Professionals who treat intravenous drug-using clients in public health clinics, methadone programs, and other settings should routinely provide educational counseling to current drug users on the risks associated with sharing needles and on the need to adopt reduced-risk sexual practices as discussed earlier. Several investigators have described programs to educate drug users concerning the risks of needle sharing and ways to clean needles prior to use (Feldman & Biernacki, 1987; Sotheran, *et al.*, 1987). However, sharing needles is common and ritualized, especially in the low-SES intravenous drug-user subculture (Lieb, *et al.*, 1987). Because the efficacy of AIDS risk-behavior-change efforts for clients who continue to use intravenous drugs is unestablished, and because persons currently addicted to injectable drugs are a difficult population to counsel with respect to making behavior change so long as they remain addicted, the most desirable therapy goal is undoubtedly involvement of the client in a treatment program for his or her drug addiction.

3.2.3. Limitations of Information Provision in Promoting Risk-Behavior Change

Counseling that consists solely of providing clients with information about means to reduce AIDS exposure risk assumes that this information can be readily put into practice. At times, this assumption is accurate. Some individuals seem able to modify their own behavior quite easily and reduce high-risk practices with little outside assistance. However, information alone may be insufficient to promote meaningful change in risk behavior, especially when that behavior is immediately reinforcing, when it is well established, and when negative consequences of the activity are temporally distant or uncertain. Many cigarette smokers continue to use tobacco, obese people continue to overeat, sedentary persons continue to remain physically inactive, and problem drinkers maintain alcohol abuse patterns even though they are cognitively aware of the long-range health threats posed by these practices. Because sex is a powerful motive and because sexual practices are maintained by past experiences, immediacy of gratification, reinforcement by fantasies, and, often, interpersonal influence or coercion, one would suspect that sexual activities are relatively difficult to change through information-provision alone. Research examining the impact of programs to prevent teenage pregnancy indicates that while information concerning pregnancy and birth control methods results in increased knowledge about contraception, information-provision alone has little impact on actual likelihood of pregnancy and sexual activity (Lance, 1975; Zuckerman, Tushup, & Finner, 1976).

In a recent study, the authors (Kelly, St. Lawrence, Brasfield, & Hood, 1987) recruited a volunteer sample of 100 men with long-standing patterns of homosexual behavior. Participants in the study had a mean age of 30.1 years, 96% were high school graduates, 88% were white and 12% were black or Hispanic, and 74% were employed full time. Most participants (73%) reported exclusively homosexual preferences, while the remainder also indicated some degree of heterosexual interest. All lived in a city with a metropolitan population of 400,000 and moderate AIDS prevalence.

Participants in the study were administered a 33-item, objective-format AIDS Risk Knowledge Test, which tapped the respondents' practical understanding about steps that can be taken to reduce AIDS risk, including the identification of high-risk practices, methods to lessen the likelihood of HIV exposure, and common misconceptions about HIV transmission. The measure's content and response scoring were based upon the findings of risk factor studies of AIDS (cf. Blattner et al., 1985; Groopman, Mayer, et al., 1985; Marmor et al., 1982; Melbye et al., 1984). Participants also completed a questionnaire to elicit detailed information about their sexual activities over the previous 12-month period, including number of different sexual partners and frequency of various specific high- and lower-risk sexual activities with those partners. The subjects varied considerably in their risk activity levels. The number of sexual partners over the past 12 months ranged from 0 to 200, and a wide range of sexual practices were reported.

In order to examine the relationship between cognitive AIDS risk knowledge and actual risk behavior, Pearson product-moment coefficients were calculated between subjects' risk knowledge scores and each assessed risk behavior. AIDS risk knowledge was not statistically related to the frequency of such high-risk practices as unprotected anal or oral intercourse as either the insertive or receptive partner, oral–anal contact, "fisting," and total number of different sexual partners, or to the frequency of lower-risk practices such as intercourse using condoms and nonpenetrative sexual activities. In addition, multiple regression analyses revealed that the frequencies of all sexual practice activities, when examined simultaneously, failed to predict subjects' cognitive knowledge about AIDS risk. At least for this sample of persons, information about AIDS risk bore no significant relationship to the frequency of actually engaging in high- or lower-risk sexual activities over the past 1-year period.

Subjects in the Kelly, St. Lawrence, Brasfield, and Hood (1987) study were males who had generally long-standing histories of well-established sexual behavior and who lived in a geographical area with only moderate AIDS prevalence and fatalities. Persons living in cities where AIDS prevalence is very high, and where many AIDS patients are personally known, may be more likely to change their own risk behavior in response to prevention messages because the threat of the disease is more salient. In addition, persons who do not yet have highly established and reinforced sexual activity patterns may find it easier to adopt reduced-risk conduct following informational counseling alone. However, the Kelly, St. Lawrence, Brasfield, and Hood (1987) findings indicate that knowledge about AIDS risk alone is not always sufficient to produce meaningful change in actual high-risk sexual behavior. While the study demonstrated this finding with a sample of homosexual males, there is little reason to suspect that different results would occur if sexually active heterosexuals were studied.

3.3. BEHAVIOR-CHANGE COUNSELING

Beyond simply providing at-risk individuals with information about high-risk practices and lower-risk alternatives, AIDS-prevention counseling can make use of more structured behavioral intervention principles to actively assist persons in reducing their risk of becoming exposed to HIV infection. The objective of such intervention is to help individuals put into practice the prevention strategies suggested in counseling or by educational materials. Persons who might benefit from more active behavioral guidance are those who are knowledgeable about AIDS risk practices but have difficulty curtailing or eliminating those sexual activities. Examples are clients who engage in unprotected intercourse with multiple partners, are worried about AIDS and seek assistance concerning it, but are not able to consistently alter their risk patterns.

In an effort to identify why people may fail to put into practice reduced-risk behavior, several studies have compared on psychological and behavioral dimensions gay men who have adopted safer sex practices with those who continue to engage in risky activities (McKusick *et al.*, 1987; Siegel *et al.*, 1987; Stall *et al.*, 1986). While the specific assessed variables differ somewhat across studies, factors associated with changes in the direction of reduced-risk behavior include beliefs that one is capable of making recommended changes ("personal efficacy"), depression, level of agreement with risk-reduction guidelines, ability to hold a visual image of the physical deterioration caused by AIDS, and perceived emotional support. Denial of the virulence of the AIDS epidemic and the frequent use of drugs and alcohol preceding sex were associated with continued high-risk conduct. Younger people were more likely to continue risky practices than older people, and persons who had primary relationships were more likely to engage in high-risk practices (McKusick et. al., 1987; Siegel et al., 1987). Such findings have led a number of researchers to conclude that risk-behavior-change interventions should include attention to social and psychological factors that can facilitate the consistent adoption of safer conduct. In addition to AIDS risk knowledge, these factors include perceived personal efficacy in successfully changing risky sexual behaviors, the development of methods to control high-risk sexual impulses, and negotiating with environmental social supports that facilitate reduced-risk life-styles (Bartlett, Rabin, Taggart, Bandemer, & Bellonti, 1987).

In a recent project, the authors and members of their research team (Kelly, St. Lawrence, Hood, & Brasfield, 1987) conducted a prevention program for 104 apparently healthy homosexual men who were concerned about AIDS and who engaged in risk activities that would result in their eventual exposure to the virus or transmission of it to others. The program consisted of 12 group training sessions to assist participants in reducing their levels of risk activity. Because there have been few empirical reports concerning prevention counseling approaches of this kind, the training program will be discussed here in detail. Participants in this project were groups of gay men at risk for HIV infection, but a similar intervention format is relevant for individual clients and for heterosexual clients who are at risk for exposure to AIDS owing to their sexual activities.

Recruitment of participants for the prevention program (called "Project Aries," an acronym for AIDS Risk Intervention Series) was accomplished by placing recruitment posters in gay bars, distributing pamphlets to bar patrons, and making brochures about the project available to physicians, college campus organizations, and persons voluntarily requesting HIV antibody testing at health department sites. Because the project was developed with the support and endorsement of gay community organization leaders, it was perceived positively in the gay community. The team conducting the project met occasionally in community settings, including bars and persons' homes, to discuss the program with potential participants and establish visibility and trust. Confidentiality safeguards were always stressed to interested persons.

Participants in the Kelly, St. Lawrence, Hood, and Brasfield (1987) project were administered a number of risk-behavior measures, including objective questionnaires assessing their sexual and drug activities over the preceding 4- and 12-month periods; self-monitoring records of sexual activities occurring over a 6-week period; self-report inventories of depression, anxiety, and health locus of control; an objective measure of knowledge about AIDS risk practices; and a measure of behavioral assertiveness skill during role-plays in which a confederate simulated verbal attempts to coerce high-risk sexual activities. Following assessments, participants were randomly assigned to either an immediate experimental intervention or a waiting-list control group. Participants in the intervention program were subdivided into smaller groups of 8 to 20 persons each in order to facilitate the training process.

Over the course of 12 meetings, participants were first provided with information about AIDS, HIV transmission, and sexual practices high or low in transmission risk. This presentation stressed that persons unexposed to HIV should remain unexposed, that persons who may have already been exposed should avoid reexposure, and that sexually active persons should accept responsibility for protecting both themselves and their partners by refraining from any activities that could pose risk to either. The material presented was similar to that discussed earlier in this chapter. Following this educational phase, the group sessions directed attention to self-management training, assertion training, and establishing relationship and life-style supports conducive to reduced risk. The purpose of the intervention was not to redirect the sexual preference of the participants or to promote total celibacy; neither goal would be realistic or appropriate for persons with well-established homosexual behavior histories. Rather, the objective was to help participants decrease high-risk sexual behavior with multiple, casual partners and encourage the adoption of reduced-risk conduct in the context of stable relationships.

3.3.1. Self-Management Training

The inability to reduce high-risk behavior patterns, whether they involve high-risk sexual practices, unsafe contacts with casual or multiple partners, or frequenting sex-oriented settings where high-risk activity often occurs, may reflect difficulties in self-management, especially when the individual is knowledgeable of AIDS risk and wishes to curtail high-risk aspects of his behavior but has trouble doing so. Such patterns often produce anxiety and worry after risky behavior takes place, but unless the individual can exert behavioral controls preceding the encounters, he or she will remain at risk.

In the Kelly, St. Lawrence, Hood, and Brasfield (1987) project, each participant generated a list of recent situations where he engaged in high-risk activities. Participants were guided in identifying antecedents to those events, including the setting where each risky encounter occurred or was arranged, any intoxicant or substance use preceding the high-risk event, the participant's own mood before the encounter, the nature of the participant's cognitive intentions prior to the event (to assess whether the high-risk encounter was actively planned or was anticipated), and any sexual fantasies that may have either preceded or followed each encounter. As expected, participants differed considerably in the specific antecedent "triggers" for their high-risk behavior, but all men were able to identify personal risk antecedents.

During the sessions on self-management, each participant was taught behavioral self-management techniques that involved rearranging the environment to decrease the probability of risk behavior's occurring. Examples included taking alternate driving routes to avoid settings conducive to high-risk casual sexual behavior, going to bars with friends rather than alone, or drinking less if intoxication was an antecedent of past risky behavior. The format of this training was modeled after self-management approaches used to help individuals reduce other kinds of maladaptive activity (cf. Blittner, Goldberg, & Merbaum, 1978; Brigham, 1978; Miller & Foy, 1981). Because gay males exposed to erotic educational materials depicting safer-sex practices reduce their levels of risky behavior (Quadland, Shattls, Schuman, & Jacobs, 1987), participants were trained to alter fantasies in order to shape themselves from images of high-risk sexual practices to fantasizing instead about low-risk erotic behavior. Assignments were made to practice self-management skills during each week between sessions. Individuals were also reinforced by the group leaders and other participants for reports of successfully avoiding high-risk antecedents, and group members were taught to reinforce themselves, as well as any sexual partners, for lower-risk conduct.

3.3.2. Assertion Training

Many project participants reported difficulty refusing pressures from partners to engage in high-risk practices. These difficulties were reflected by unassertive performance during the pretraining assessment role-plays in which a confederate simulated verbal attempts to coerce high-risk conduct. Consequently, several group sessions focused on assertiveness training. The procedures employed were adapted from standard traditional assertion training research and included instruction, modeling, and behavior rehearsal (role playing) followed by feedback (Hersen, Eisler, Miller, Johnson, & Pinkston, 1973; Hersen, Kazdin, Bellack, & Turner, 1979; Kelly, 1982). The objective of this intervention component was to increase participants' skill and comfort in firmly declining pressures from others to engage in a high-risk practice, suggesting a lower-risk alternative (if a sexual encounter was taking place), and declining propositions for unwanted casual sexual encounters. In group sessions, participants practiced role-play situations requiring assertiveness in order to decline a high-risk coercion and were instructed to apply the same skills when coercive situations occurred between sessions. In addition, the participants role-played how they would initiate discussion with a partner expressing their intention to engage only in lower-risk behavior. It was stressed that such discussion, when initiated well ahead of the time of sexual activity, could serve to clarify health interest with a partner and to establish "ground rules" for remaining at low risk.

3.3.3. Life-Style Issues

For persons who are not celibate, steady relationships characterized by consistent lower-risk practices and mutual health concern place an individual at lower AIDS risk than having anonymous or casual sexual contacts characterized by high-risk practices and limited interest in the future well-being of the partners. Most participants in the project reported desiring steady relationships but also reported having difficulty initiating or maintaining them.

In order to assist group members in establishing life-styles that support lower-risk behavior, discussion focused on the benefits of developing relationships based on nonsexual social "dating," rather than immediate sex-partner seeking, and delaying sexual activity until mutual understanding concerning the need for lower-risk practices had been established between partners. The authors are aware that the goal of helping gay men to develop steady relationships with same-sex partners may be seen as controversial by some persons. However, as discussed earlier, it is critical that AIDS-prevention counseling be practical, effective, and nonprejudicial, and that it take into account the life-styles of the individuals being counseled.

Finally, participants were encouraged to identify and involve themselves in socially supportive activities that would serve to maintain self-pride, self-esteem, and reduced-risk conduct. Some of these activities were unstructured and informal, such as spending increased time in socializing with friends. Others entailed participation in community activities that could reinforce a sense of pride in oneself and others, such as involvement in AIDS-prevention fund-raising efforts and volunteer work in health clinics and community programs.

3.3.4. Program Effectiveness

The effectiveness of the Kelly, St. Lawrence, Hood, and Brasfield (1987) project was assessed by examining change on the various risk measures from pre- to postintervention points for program participants compared with change on the measures over the same time period for waiting-list control group subjects. These analyses confirmed the effectiveness of the intervention. Although the intervention and control groups did not differ from one another at the preintervention point, program participants engaged in significantly fewer high-risk sexual behaviors with fewer different partners than control group subjects after the intervention. Specifically, intervention participants reported less-frequent occurrences of unprotected anal intercourse, had fewer different sexual partners, and less frequently visited casual sex-oriented "cruising" areas such as pornographic bookstores and parks than did control group members. The mean proportion of sexual activities characterized by safer sex practices (using condoms or engaging in practices that did not involve fluid exchange) was significantly higher for persons who had participated in the program, and participants achieved significantly higher scores on the test of AIDS risk knowledge. When role-plays of performance in situations requiring assertiveness to resist high-risk sexual coercions were rated, participants in the intervention program were found to be more appropriately assertive than control group subjects. Taken together, these data confirmed that participation in the group intervention produced significant increases in AIDS-risk knowledge and behavioral skills relevant to risk reduction and, most important, resulted in substantially reduced high-risk conduct.

3.3.5. Implications for Individuals and Group Counseling

The prevention counseling model evaluated by Kelly, St. Lawrence, Hood, and Brasfield (1987) is based on the assumption that well-established, long-standing patterns of high-risk behavior not readily changed by the provision of AIDS educational information alone can be reduced if specific behavior change guidance is also offered. Because the intervention described here combined multiple components (self-management assistance to avoid high-risk conduct, group support, assertion training to help participants initiate discussion with partners about lower-risk practices and to resist high-risk coercions, and attention to life-style, relationship, social, and self-pride issues), it is not possible to determine which of these training areas most contributed to reductions in high-risk conduct. We suspect that different intervention elements were most salient for different individuals. Persons whose high-risk activities are preceded by intoxication or visiting a "cruising" setting may benefit most from self-management approaches that emphasize ways to avoid or handle differently these risk antecedents. Persons who are knowledgeable about safer practices but are unable to resist pressures from partners to engage in high-risk behavior may benefit most from assertion training. Many participants in the study reported that attention to the development and maintenance of steady relationships with a partner also contributed to lower-risk conduct. When counseling an individual client, it is advisable to determine why high-risk behavior occurs and to then tailor the counseling intervention to address those factors that are most responsible for risk behavior (Bartlett *et al.*, 1987). An ongoing assessment of the client's risk behavior, such as self-monitored client recordings of the frequency of high- and low-risk sexual practices, number of different partners, and mood, substance use, and setting antecedents of any high-risk behavior, can provide a useful means to evaluate the effectiveness of the counseling intervention.

The Kelly, St. Lawrence, Hood, and Brasfield (1987) project had, as its participants, groups of sexually active gay men who were at risk for AIDS owing to the nature of the sexual practices in which they engaged. As discussed earlier, homosexual or bisexual males are at risk only if they engage in practices that permit the efficient transmission of HIV. Many gay men have already modified their behavior so as to reduce AIDS risk (Joseph *et al.*, 1987). However, gay men who have not engaged in or men who still periodically engage in high-risk practices should be counseled as intensively as possible to behave in a less risky manner.

Finally, while the project described in this chapter intervened with homosexual males, the same intervention components are likely to prove relevant for encouraging behavior change of heterosexual clients at risk for HIV infection. Lack of accurate information about AIDS risk behaviors, denial of personal vulnerability to AIDS, difficulties in the self-management of risky behavior, inability to resist sexual coercion, difficulty establishing steady relationships is characterized by low-risk behavior, and a paucity of social supports conducive to self-pride and self-esteem can be responsible for high-risk life-styles among some heterosexuals. With minor variations in specific content, the same intervention approaches described here for gay men may prove useful for at-risk heterosexuals.

Behavioral Interventions at a Community Level

Individual and small group counseling efforts are appropriate and necessary when assisting help-seeking clients who are at risk for AIDS. However, in spite of the media attention that AIDS receives and the fear that AIDS can engender, it is not likely that most persons at risk for the syndrome will seek out individual risk-behavior-change assistance even from care-providers who are trusted. The stigma associated with acknowledging that one is at risk for AIDS and concerns regarding potential breaches in confidentiality make it unlikely that large numbers of persons will initiate requests for assistance in reducing their personal AIDS risk. Many investigators in the primary prevention area have also noted that traditional mental health service provision systems that require persons to "come to" therapy may be useful for a small number of help-seeking individuals but are generally ineffective in promoting behavior change on the wide-scale level needed for community prevention (Fredericksen, Solomon, & Brehony, 1984; Rosen & Solomon, 1985). Even if all persons at risk for AIDS were willing to seek out assistance to reduce their exposure risk, traditional mental health and therapy-based counseling systems could not possibly accommodate them (Solomon, 1986). Many public health clinics now have waiting lists of weeks or months for persons who simply seek routine, voluntary HIV-antibody testing, which requires much less time than comprehensive counseling. Given that there are still relatively few professionals, organizations, or clinics able to deal capably with the needs of individual AIDS at-risk or AIDS-affected persons, it is evident that primary prevention efforts must be community-based and wide scale if they are to be effective.

Partly because AIDS prevention is such a new area, there have been few empirical studies evaluating the effectiveness of specific community AIDS risk-reduction approaches. In addition to the recency of the problem, research on prevention is hindered by the fact that AIDS often does not develop until years after the activities causing exposure to the HIV virus took place. Therefore, it is not possible to implement a program and determine whether it reduces the number of actual new AIDS cases until years have passed. While it is theoretically possible to more quickly assess the impact of prevention programs by observing changes in the prevalence of HIV infection (as reflected by HIV-antibody-positive rates) in the population targeted for prevention, sampling, logistical, and ethical issues involved in large-scale antibody testing often limit the feasibility of this approach to evaluating prevention efforts. It is more practical, albeit less direct, to attempt to experimentally establish by survey whether prevention efforts change people's accurate knowledge of AIDS risk behaviors or their reported frequency of engaging in high-risk practices. In addition, change in AIDS risk behavior can be indirectly inferred by changes in more readily measurable activities that are correlated with AIDS risk practices. Some studies have inferred a reduction in the frequency of AIDS risk behavior by a decrease in the number of cases of reportable sexually transmitted diseases such as gonorrhea or syphilis in certain cities (Golubjatnikov, Pfister, & Tillotson, 1983; Schechter et al., 1984). Because these diseases are transmitted in the same way as HIV infection, reductions in the incidence of "traditional" sexually transmitted diseases can serve as a rough measure of AIDS risk behavior change. Sales of condoms in a geographical area may also indirectly reflect gross changes in the population's awareness of AIDS risk.

In spite of the difficulties involved in measuring the impact of community AIDS programs, empirical research on this topic is clearly needed. Without evaluative research, it will be impossible to determine what types of educational and risk-behavior-change approaches are most effective for what populations. Further, there is a need for wide-scale dissemination of both detailed prevention program descriptions and data concerning their efficacy. Especially in the case of AIDS, where the timely implementation of wide-scale prevention programs is essential, it is dangerous and time-inefficient for agencies and organizations in various cities to develop programs independently without an awareness of the success or pitfalls of similar efforts elsewhere.

In this chapter, some approaches to AIDS prevention at a community level will be considered. Because there have been few empirical outcome studies of these prevention approaches, their impact has also not yet been conclusively established. Nonetheless, given the AIDS-prevention programs that have already been developed and research already conducted on primary prevention/risk-reduction methods in other health-related areas, it is possible to identify mechanisms for promoting reduced-risk conduct. Effective prevention must take into account the need to (1) provide accurate information on AIDS high-risk practices and lower-risk alternatives on a wide scale, with the specific content of messages tailored to the targeted population; (2) provide environmental cues and prompts so that people remember the educational messages and actually adopt the behavior suggested in them; and (3) provide environmental/social supports that serve to maintain lower-risk conduct until it becomes well established.

4.1. INFORMATIONAL AND EDUCATIONAL MESSAGES

Although the topic of AIDS prevention is new, there is a well-developed literature on characteristics of public health messages that best educate persons concerning threats to their well-being. This literature indicates that effective health/behavior-change-education messages include explicit information indicating that the severity of the potential illness is great, that the individual receiving the message is susceptible to the illness, that behavior change can be effected to reduce the likelihood of illness, and that the relative benefits of behavior change are greater than the costs. In addition, health-promotion messages are most effective when they provide information on the specific behavior change needed to reduce risk, offer a cognitive rationale for the reasons that those specific behavior changes reduce the risk of illness, and provide encouragement for making health-related changes (cf. Leventhal, Safer, & Panagis, 1983; Siegel *et al.*, 1986).

In the case of AIDS prevention, educational messages have often been conveyed through brochures and pamphlets developed by national and "mainstream" public health agencies, state and local health agencies, AIDS task forces, and gay community organizations. The specific content and tone of AIDS-prevention pamphlets vary considerably, depending upon the target readership group for the materials (e.g., gay men, intravenous drug users, heterosexuals, adolescents, and other groups) and, often, upon the traditionalism or nontraditionalism of the organizations that developed them. Siegel *et al.* (1986) reviewed 22 AIDS-prevention brochures targeted toward gay or bisexual men, examining similarities and differences in their content relative to criteria for effectiveness in public health communications. While most of the AIDS-prevention pamphlets, regardless of the organization that developed them, included communications likely to invoke in the reader a sense of threat, discussed the causes of AIDS, and provided information on high-risk sexual practices to avoid, less than half offered the reader information on why particular practices are risky. This deficit is significant because compliance with behavior-change recommendations is higher when clear rationales for change are included (Chambless & Goldstein, 1979; Orne & Wender, 1968).

Siegel *et al.* (1986) also found that AIDS-prevention brochures often lack specific, accurate descriptions of lower-risk practices and generally fail to advise the reader concerning "action-oriented" ways to put lower-risk behavior into effect. In addition, Siegel *et al.* (1986) fault many AIDS informational brochures for failing to instill in readers the belief that behavior changes can be made, for neglecting to provide positive motivational encouragement, and occasionally for offering ambiguous information that may mislead readers. For example, "reducing one's number of sexual partners," a common informational message, would afford little practical benefit if a gay male decreased from 30 different partners per year to 15 partners in a year but engaged in high-risk sexual practices with them.

On the basis of these observations, it is possible to identify several desirable characteristics of AIDS educational pamphlets, posters, or advertisements. First, educational materials should present clear information about AIDS, including why it is a serious health threat, how the virus causing it is transmitted, and why behavior change can prevent illness. High-risk practices, described in language that will be understood by the reader, are identified, along with brief explanations concerning the reasons that various practices are risky. Lower-risk alternatives are described, including concrete suggestions for putting these alternatives into practice (such as by clarifying with a sexual partner in advance the importance of safer sex practices, avoiding alcohol overuse because it often impairs judgment, or keeping condoms readily available if one may be sexually active). Finally, and as suggested by Siegel *et al.* (1986), educational messages should emphasize that risk-reduction-behavior changes can be made, will result in greater feelings of self-esteem and control over health, and represent positive steps for better protecting both oneself and others from AIDS. Before developing brochures or other written materials, AIDS-prevention educators should examine materials already in use by other organizations. This saves time and allows AIDS educators to benefit from the strengths and to address the limitations of existing materials.

Written materials on AIDS prevention are useful because they are inexpensive and can be mass-distributed or posted where targeted populations can read them. The content and language used in written materials can also be tailored to the specific populations for which they are intended. Many AIDS-prevention programs, especially in large cities, have developed different brochures for gay men, heterosexuals with multiple partners, Spanish-speaking persons, IV drug users, adolescents, and the "mainstream" general population, with educational content tailored to the targeted group. This is an appropriate strategy because information and language relevant to one group might be ineffective or inappropriate for other groups of people.

In order to have the greatest impact, written AIDS-prevention materials must reach and be read by persons at risk. Gay bars, clubs, and businesses in large cities sometimes make AIDS-prevention brochures available to their patrons, and some national magazines and newspapers with gay readerships print guidelines concerning AIDS risk reduction for their readers. Health departments and public health clinics in many cities provide brochures about AIDS to persons receiving contraception counseling or treatment for drug use and sexually transmitted diseases. Although these distribution methods for written materials on AIDS prevention are exceedingly important and necessary, they are no longer sufficient. As the population at risk for HIV infection grows to include potentially nonmonogamous heterosexuals, information-provision on a much broader scale is needed. Some colleges and universities now provide all students with AIDS educational materials, and military personnel receive prevention materials. We believe that these efforts should be expanded. Just as many gay bars and businesses have taken steps to provide educational materials for their patrons, clubs and "singles" bars oriented toward sexually active heterosexuals could serve as useful dissemination points for educational materials. Focused efforts are especially needed in low-income black and Hispanic communities, both because racial minorities account for a disproportionately large number of AIDS cases (Selik & Rogers, 1987) and because increased heterosexual transmission is likely from HIV-infected intravenous drug users concentrated in impoverished urban areas to their sexual partners.

Some European and Scandinavian countries are initiating educational efforts on an even larger scale. In Great Britain, AIDS-prevention information has been mailed to all households in the country (Pickles & Bond, 1987). Many nations now sponsor AIDS educational messages in both the print and broadcast media. While the content of such wide-scale messages is primarily limited to alerting citizens about AIDS and offering general prevention recommendations, they no doubt raise levels of public awareness of AIDS. This function alone is of importance, especially in the heterosexual community, where individuals with multiple partners who are at risk for AIDS may not currently perceive themselves as even vulnerable to the disease.

4.1.1. Limitations of Written Materials for AIDS Prevention

Print materials such as pamphlets, brochures, or advertisements are necessary to educate persons about ways to reduce exposure risk. On the other hand, brochure-based information alone may be insufficient to produce meaningful, wide-scale change in actual risk behavior. For educational objectives to be met, individuals at risk for AIDS must initiate the steps of picking up, reading, and attending closely to the information presented in pamphlets or brochures. While the time and effort needed to do so are not great, there are few data to indicate how many individuals at high risk really do spontaneously read pamphlets or recall the most critical information contained in them. Research in other areas of health promotion does not support the contention that pamphlets are a highly effective way to instill the motivation to make changes in long-standing risk behavior. Patterns of cigarette smoking, problem drinking, drug abuse, breast self-examination, and cardiovascular fitness do not change substantially in a population even when brief written informational materials on behavior change are made available (McAlister, 1984; Ockene & Camic, 1985; Swain & Stekel, 1981). As noted in Chapter 3, pamphlet-based information about contraception provided to teenagers appears to have little impact on either their patterns of sexual activity or their likelihood of becoming pregnant (Lance, 1975; Zuckerman *et al.*, 1976). Thus, while the distribution of printed informational materials represents an efficient and necessary aspect of AIDS education, other educational vehicles are also needed to promote reduced-risk conduct at a community level.

4.1.2. Additional Means of Public Education

Public opinion research shows that people gain a great deal of knowledge about events taking place around them and form opinions about those events as a result of personal communication—talking—with others (Kleppner, Russell, & Verrill, 1983; Kotler, 1983). Information presented in the context of talking or discussion has a number of advantages relative to printed materials alone. Discussion-based presentation of information provides an opportunity for the listener to ask questions and have those questions clarified. Motivational encouragement to put information into practice is often more easily afforded in conversational exchanges than in brief printed materials. And, when the person presenting information is perceived as credible, sympathetic, and similar to the listener, the information conveyed is high in influence and believability (Kleppner *et al.*, 1983).

In a number of cities and states, health organizations concerned with AIDS prevention have sponsored educational programs conducted in settings where risk-group members meet and socialize. The Ohio Department of Health has a professional staff member (Buck Harris) who regularly visits gay bars in the state and presents programs on risk reduction to bar patrons. These presentations, which include standard risk-reduction information, also permit the audience to ask questions and to discuss ways to put into practice the information that is presented. This approach is useful because it places resource persons in a community setting rather than requiring persons at risk to initiate information-seeking efforts.

Other programs have further extended this community-based education model by providing AIDS educational training to "key" persons who are already established in the community. An example of this approach is conducting AIDS educational programs for bartenders so that they can, in turn, convey the same information to others with whom they interact naturally on a day-to-day basis (Kelly & St. Lawrence, 1987b; Solomon, in press). By identifying and providing risk information to persons who are influential with others in their natural social networks, it is possible to set in motion a process of peer education (Kelly & St. Lawrence, 1987b). However, for this model to be maximally effective, it is necessary not only to provide risk-reduction information to key people in a community but also to train them in ways to actively educate others with whom they have contact.

In an innovative "grass roots" approach to community AIDS education, the "Stop AIDS" organization in San Francisco has implemented a program in which staff members or trained volunteers conduct AIDS education sessions in social settings, including private homes. This model, already employed successfully to teach women breast self-examination skills (Strauss, Solomon, Costanza, Worden, & Foster, 1987; Worden *et al.*, 1987), is a potentially useful way to promote behavior change when the health subject is sufficiently embarrassing or stigmatizing that individuals would be reluctant to seek out assistance or information in more public ways. With respect to AIDS, groups of friends and acquaintances interested in learning more about risk reduction are invited to an informal gathering by a person organizing the session, and an AIDS educator leads an informational discussion concerning risk reduction. Although this "Tupperware party" approach to AIDS education appears cumbersome, it has been well received. As we will discuss shortly, such educational strategies can be effective not only in imparting information but also for establishing supports and norms favoring reduced-risk conduct within individuals' natural peer networks.

Because AIDS has taken its greatest toll in large American cities, the most established prevention programs have also been focused in those areas. However, as the health crisis expands, aggressive prevention campaigns are needed in other geographical areas. Gay and bisexually active men in small cities and rural areas are at imminent risk but are more difficult to reach with prevention messages than are homosexuals in large cities. Because many smaller cities still have had a relatively small number of AIDS cases, gay men in those cities may not perceive a sufficient personal threat from AIDS to motivate substantial change in risk behavior. By the time actual AIDS cases increase enough to cause personal alarm, the prevalence of HIV infection will also be so high that primary prevention will be much less effective. Prevention efforts in smaller cities are also often hindered by the lack of formal AIDS-prevention resources or centers and the more hidden and "closeted" nature of the gay communities in them.

To a substantial extent, similar barriers exist to community AIDS-prevention efforts among intravenous drug users. A small proportion of

IV drug users are identifiable because they are in treatment programs, methadone maintenance centers, or the criminal justice system. However, most intravenous drug users are "hidden" in a community and, therefore, are difficult to specifically target in prevention campaigns. The illegal nature of drug use, the fact that users are addicted to drugs, and distrustful relations with traditional public health authorities further complicate AIDS-prevention efforts with this population.

Treatment to eliminate addiction is clearly the intervention of choice for intravenous drug users. However, outcome studies often do not demonstrate long-term success following detoxification treatment for chronic drug addiction (Alford, 1981), and the number of available openings in no-cost or low-cost drug treatment facilities is far less than the need. Because HIV infection rates among urban intravenous drug users in some large cities are high (Drucker & Vermund, 1987; Marlink *et al.*, 1987), because most drug users share or reuse needles (Abdul-Quader *et al.*, 1987), and because IV drug users constitute a major transmission "bridge" for HIV infection to the general heterosexual community, AIDS prevention is closely linked to improved success and increased availability of drug treatment and methadone maintenance programs for addicts. In addition, interventions that prevent intravenous drug use or interrupt patterns of occasional IV drug use before chronic addiction occurs can also have major impact on AIDS primary prevention.

Efforts to curtail the spread of AIDS among current intravenous drug users and from IV drug users to their sexual contacts emphasize risk education. To discourage the sharing of HIV-contaminated syringes, some community-based programs instruct drug users in methods to disinfect needles prior to reuse (Feldman & Biernacki, 1987; Watters, 1987). Such interventions often utilize addicts, former addicts, or other staff credible to the IV drug user population as field intervention agents. Some authorities believe needle sharing among addicts occurs because clean needles are unavailable; in most states, syringes can be purchased only by prescription. In several countries, clean syringes are now provided to addicts, sometimes in exchange for used ones, in an effort to discourage needle reuse (Buning, 1987; Wodak *et al.*, 1987). Similar proposals in the United States have generally met with political resistance on the grounds that distributing needles to addicts may promote, or be perceived as promoting, intravenous drug use. Unfortunately, little outcome research evaluating the efficacy of various approaches for discouraging needle sharing and for encouraging safer sex practices by intravenous drug users has yet been conducted. It is likely that AIDS prevention with this population will need to combine (1) efforts to better prevent young persons at risk for IV drug use from becoming addicted, (2) improved availability of effective detoxification and/or methadone maintenance treatment programs, especially for those urban poor who are currently addicted, and (3) community-based programs to educate and encourage addicts either to use clean needles or to disinfect needles before reuse.

4.1.3. AIDS Risk Education for Adolescents

Prevention efforts for sexually active adults and for persons in current AIDS risk groups are needed immediately to curtail the spread of AIDS. For the longer term, it is equally critical to educate children and adolescents concerning AIDS. If young people are provided with current information about AIDS before they become sexually active, they will be in a better position to protect themselves from AIDS and HIV infection.

Many junior high schools and high schools are now considering or are implementing AIDS education and occasionally conduct educational presentations for students (Komada & O'Donnell, 1987; Walton, 1987). The objective of AIDS education for older children and adolescents does not differ from the aims of educational efforts for other populations. Providing factual and clear information about the syndrome, dispelling misconceptions about casual transmission, conveying accurate information about high-risk behaviors, and advising persons of ways to lessen exposure risk are fundamental objectives for all educational programs.

However, there are special issues that bear on AIDS education efforts, particularly at the secondary school level. The purpose of teaching persons about AIDS early in their lives is to reduce the likelihood that they will later begin to engage in activities that could pose a health risk. This means that the information conveyed to young people not only must be accurate at the time it is taught but also most anticipate the health crisis and risk behaviors that will be salient several years into the future. Some of the more "narrow" risk messages concerning AIDS need to be replaced by more general cautions and information that will not quickly become outdated. For example, by stressing that homosexual males with multiple partners are at greatest risk for AIDS, educators may create the impression that heterosexuals are not at risk. By the time that most school-age

young people become sexually active, heterosexuals with multiple partners will also be at significant risk for AIDS. In similar fashion, engaging
in unprotected anal intercourse is one of the strongest risk factors in the
histories of homosexual males currently diagnosed with AIDS. However,
the changing epidemiology of the health crisis suggests that any kind of
unprotected intercourse between nonexclusive partners, whether
homosexual or heterosexual, will carry potential risk. AIDS educators
who conduct programs for young people face the challenging tasks of
both describing accurately the current state of our knowledge about the
illness and presenting prevention recommendations that will remain
salient several years in the future.

Just as few physicians, psychologists, social workers, or other
professionals were originally trained to counsel persons at risk for AIDS
or persons already affected by the illness, few teachers have had training
in AIDS education. This means that secondary-level educators without
expertise in AIDS prevention will require access to suitable teaching
resource materials and should establish cooperative relationships with
AIDS authorities in their area who can advise as to the content and
development of educational programs. Because public misconceptions
about AIDS are so common and because the need for clearly presented,
factual information is so great, it is imperative that AIDS education
programs be developed with careful attention to accuracy.

AIDS is a controversial topic, and the issue of how best to inform
young people about steps that can be taken to prevent AIDS has proven
controversial in much the same way as school-based sex education. Some
conservative educators maintain that young people should be taught that
only chastity and monogamy assure protection against sexually transmitted HIV infection. Pragmatic and public-health-oriented educators argue
that young persons should be provided with practical information on
how to reduce AIDS risk in the event they do not maintain a single
lifelong monogamous relationship. It is likely that AIDS education
programs in different schools will vary in the extent to which they
advocate the values of chastity or monogamy, just as sex education
programs vary in their handling of these values. However, given the
magnitude and seriousness of the AIDS health crisis, it seems to the
authors irresponsible not to also provide specific risk-reduction
recommendations, such as using condoms, for persons who do become
sexually active.

4.2. PROVISION OF CUES TO ADOPT LOWER-RISK
BEHAVIOR

It is a well-established principle that imediate consequences tend to exert a stronger influence over behavior than long-delayed consequences, even if those delayed consequences are health threatening. This principle has been used to explain why a variety of maladaptive health behavior patterns, such as smoking, overeating, and alcohol or chemical abuse, are maintained even when the individual who engages in them "knows" the patterns are hazardous. Especially when persons already have well-established patterns of smoking, overeating, and substance abuse, information about the risks of these activities and brief instructions to change the patterns are often ineffective in producing significant behavior change. Consequently, intervention programs for such problems often incorporate additional mechanisms to promote change. These mechanisms include frequent prompts or reminders to refrain from the health-risk activity, efforts to bring awareness of the long-term negative health outcome "closer" to the risk-temptation activity, and the provision of models, supports, and reinforcement of reduced-risk conduct (McAlister, 1984; Ockene & Camic, 1985; Sackett, et al., 1975; Swain & Stekel, 1981).

With respect to AIDS, the feared health consequence—development of illness—may not occur until many years after risk activities and initial exposure to the HIV virus take place. In contrast, the sexual activities that carry AIDS risk are immediately reinforcing for many individuals, are long-standing, and were not in the past generally associated with the potential for causing a serious health threat. This suggests that isolated AIDS educational messages, whether provided in a brochure, article, or presentation, are not likely to be sufficient to promote the consistent adoption of lower-risk conduct. As discussed in Chapter 3, cognitive knowledge about AIDS risk may be unrelated to actual personal risk conduct, at least in persons with a well-established history of high-risk behavior (Kelly, St. Lawrence, Brasfield, & Hood,1987). For that reason, community AIDS-prevention efforts must include behavior-change assistance mechanisms beyond simply providing brief information.

4.2.1. Prompts

One of the most basic methods to promote reduced-risk conduct is to remind persons frequently about the importance of taking consistent prevention steps. Prompts can be given in many ways, but the most efficient prompts at a community level are often visual or media-based. Bars and businesses in the gay communities of some large cities participate in well-developed prompt campaigns to promote lower-risk behavior. Posters with such messages as "People who care play safe," "Even if your partner is uninformed about AIDS, it's still your responsibility to keep things safe," "Real men use condoms, " and "Be proud of yourself, play safe" are displayed in some settings. While these messages have been most extensively used in the gay community, similar prompts to avoid intravenous drug use and prompts oriented to prevention among heterosexuals are also necessary.

There has been no research on the types of prompt messages that are most likely to influence community behavior with respect to AIDS. However, studies of media influence indicate that messages are more effective when they are memorable and likely to "stand out" and be noticed, when they are relatively brief, and when they suggest a prescriptive positive course of action. Presentations of message variations or the presentation of prompts in different modalities (such as written, graphic, or audio) are more effective than repetitions of the same message in the same presentation mode (Bovee & Arens, 1986). Prompts serve as brief cues to remember and to apply previously learned information about AIDS risk reduction. Consequently, prompt messages should follow or should accompany more specific risk-education campaigns. Reminding at-risk persons to "practice safety" carries little impact unless members of the target population already understand what this means and how to accomplish it.

Prompt message posters or signs can be placed in settings frequented by persons at risk for AIDS, such as gay bars, heterosexual "singles" bars, public health clinics, college campuses, and inner-city areas with high concentrations of intravenous drug users. The prevention prompt messages can then be tailored, in content and language, to the risk group most likely to see them. Wide-scale mass-media messages on television, on radio, and in the print media, as well as AIDS-prevention prompts to adolescents in school, are also needed to reinforce the importance of adopting lower-risk behavior. Even minimal steps in this direction, such as broadcast media advertisements for condoms, have created controversy in some segments of the community. However, as the spread of AIDS continues, the preservation of public health will clearly have to take precedence over lesser concerns about decorum and taste.

4.2.2. Increasing the Perceived Salience of the AIDS Health Threat

As discussed earlier, AIDS develops long after the time when an individual engages in activities that produce HIV infection. Consequently, AIDS may not be perceived as a threat even by persons who are at risk for the syndrome. In order to motivate attention to prevention messages and promote the adoption of lower-risk conduct patterns, persons at risk for AIDS must perceive themselves to be threatened and must then believe that personal behavior change can alter their risk.

Knowing friends or acquaintances with AIDS is a stark reminder of the health crisis. When individuals personally know AIDS patients and people who have died of AIDS, and when those patients are perceived as similar to oneself, the salience of the health crisis is intensified. Although there have not been city-by-city empirical comparisons, it appears that gay men in large cities with the greatest number of AIDS cases are most likely to have reduced their frequency of engaging in high-risk sexual practices (McKusick, Horstman, & Coates, 1985). While this may be due to more focused educational campaigns in large cities, it perhaps also reflects the fact that gay men in these areas know people with AIDS and therefore perceive the threat as more imminent and personal. Further supporting this notion is the finding that being able to visually picture the physical deterioration that accompanies AIDS predicts a significant reduction in number of different sexual partners (McKusick *et al.*, 1987). Sadly, by the time that many AIDS patients are widely known and widely visible in a community, the prevalence of HIV infection among risk-group populations is also likely to already be high, lessening the potential impact of primary prevention efforts.

From a public health perspective, it would be desirable if persons with AIDS were visible and known; this would, no doubt, contribute to greater awareness of the disease and a more wide-scale perception of threat among people who do not yet perceive themselves to be at risk. Unfortunately, the stigma associated with AIDS and the potential for discrimination or ostracism are great and still lead many persons affected by the disease to keep their health status secret. Nonetheless, persons with AIDS who are willing to be publicly visible and to occupy roles that educate and sensitize others to the health threat contribute meaningfully to prevention efforts.

Media portrayals, when properly handled, can increase accurate public awareness about AIDS, alert persons to threat, correct common misconceptions, and educate the community concerning risk reduction. Feature stories that portray nongay "stereotyped" AIDS patients—including women, black and Hispanic persons, and persons from smaller communities—may serve the especially useful function of promoting greater awareness of the threat posed by AIDS to individuals at risk outside the gay communities of the largest cities.

As several investigators (Leventhal *et al.*, 1983; Siegel *et al.*, 1986) have pointed out, persons at risk for AIDS will not alter high-risk practices unless they perceive themselves to be personally vulnerable to the disease. On the other hand, prevention campaigns based only on fear are likely to prove ineffective and may carry negative repercussions. The induction of fear alone does not consistently produce change in other health-risk behaviors, including smoking or substance use (Maburn, 1982; Thompson, 1978). If individuals are overwhelmed by fear, they may feel that change is pointless or impossible to effect and that disease exposure is inevitable (Siegel *et al.*, 1986). In addition, public campaigns that emphasize only fear of AIDS can exacerbate public hysteria, creating unnecessary anxiety for persons not at risk and contributing to unwarranted discrimination for those with AIDS and HIV infection. The most useful community strategy appears to entail the induction of realistic personal fear and threat among persons who are at risk for HIV infection and the provision of educational intervention, behavior-change prompts, and support mechanisms to maintain lower-risk conduct.

4.2.3. Modeling Influences

An extensive body of literature has shown that models influence the behavior of persons observing them (Bandura, 1969; Bandura & Walters, 1963). Although models may be symbolic or may involve verbal or visual depictions of conduct, live models—other people who are perceived as realistic, similar to the observer, and likable and warm—are the most important modeling influences on human behavior. Models teach behavior to the persons observing them, but they also serve to legitimize and reinforce new standards of conduct and can demonstrate to others that behavior change can be successfully made. This concept of self-efficacy plays a role in determining whether persons at risk for AIDS make behavior changes to reduce their levels of risk. In a large sample of gay men, the belief that one was personally capable of making recommended changes to lessen AIDS exposure risk was the variable that most strongly predicted whether persons actually adopted lower-risk conduct (R.A. Coates *et al.*, 1987; McKusick *et al.*, 1987). Models who demonstrate ways to successfully cope with the threat of AIDS by reducing high-risk behavior are likely to strengthen the social appropriateness of making risk-reduction changes.

Probably because of the stigma associated with AIDS, AIDS risk groups, and AIDS risk behaviors, most messages about prevention have been delivered using impersonal communication methods, low in modeling salience, such as brochures and posters. It is still quite rare for well-known, respected, and recognizable public figures to educate people about AIDS risk practices, and it is even more rare when admired public figures, credible to persons who are at risk for AIDS, publicly discuss changes they have made in their own behavior. It is unfortunate that few well-known figures—such as athletes, entertainers, and others—have yet served as media spokespersons willing to offer specific, constructive AIDS-prevention recommendations. Because models are most influential when they are perceived as credible to the persons observing them, messages targeted to the gay adult community should be from persons well regarded by gay men. Spokespersons for messages intended primarily for racial minorities should be individuals respected in the black and Hispanic communities, while the providers of AIDS-prevention messages for adolescents are most appropriately persons already well known and respected by teenagers.

On a more personal level, peers serve as influential models, help to define standards of appropriate conduct within their social networks, and can function as credible information sources to others. To the extent that personal friends and acquaintances have altered their risk behavior, and to the extent that these changes are known to others, modeling influences are present that favor the adoption of lower-risk conduct. Because the behaviors that pose the greatest risk for HIV transmission typically occur in private and are not publicly observable to others, direct modeling of lower-risk conduct is not likely to occur. Nonetheless, if individuals who have changed risky patterns can be encouraged to discuss with peers how and why they changed their behavior, an important force to promote risk reduction can be harnessed. Examples of this approach include encouraging health-conscious gay men to discuss with their peers how and why they have altered their sexual practices, encouraging persons who use or were tempted to use intravenous drugs to discuss with other drug users the risk of AIDS, and encouraging heterosexuals who had engaged in high-risk practices with multiple partners to talk with their friends about behavior changes that they have effected.

The prevention approach requires that persons who are knowledgeable about AIDS and who have made risk-reduction behavior change become able to converse with others about sexual conduct. Given the discomfort experienced by most people when talking about sex, it may prove desirable to specifically train AIDS-knowledgeable persons in ways to initiate discussions with others about risk precautions. By not only teaching prevention to individuals who are at risk for AIDS but also specifically enlisting their assistance as behavior-change agents for others in their social networks, community prevention efforts can be multiplied and made more effective (Kelly & St. Lawrence, 1987b).

4.3. SUPPORTS FOR MAINTENANCE OF RISK-BEHAVIOR CHANGE

All available evidence indicates that the prevalence of HIV infection will continue to escalate greatly in the United States and worldwide (World Health Organization, 1987). Until biomedical research results in the development of vaccines against HIV infection or ways to biologically reduce the infectiousness of persons who carry HIV infection, persons at risk for AIDS must adopt and then consistently maintain patterns of reduced-risk conduct over extended periods of time. Transitory or inconsistent behavior change will be insufficient to protect individuals from AIDS as the prevalence of HIV infection increases and the health risks associated with even occasional occurrences of high-risk conduct become correspondingly higher.

Abstinence represents a life-style choice that some persons, both homosexual and heterosexual, have made in response to the health crisis (Hirsch & Enlow, 1984). For these individuals, reducing or eliminating anxiety concerning possible exposure to AIDS is sufficient to motivate the adoption of a completely celibate life-style.

Attempts to reduce one's number of different sexual partners and redefine the nature of sexual activities that do occur are likely to be more common responses to the threat of AIDS than permanent, lifelong celibacy. For persons accustomed to having multiple partners or casual sexual relationships, and for persons who have engaged in what are now known to be high-risk sexual practices, ongoing environmental supports may be needed to sustain new patterns of reduced-risk conduct. Although there has been no research conducted to date on the types of support that best facilitate the maintenance of low-risk behavior for AIDS, several areas merit attention.

The community intervention components discussed earlier in this chapter—including prompts or reminders concerning prevention, visible models who demonstrate to others the need for behavior-change efforts, and more frequent communication by people within natural social networks to reinforce the social acceptability of taking steps to reduce AIDS risk—are likely to help sustain reduced-risk behavior. In addition, social structures that promote the adoption of stable, health-conscious relationships are needed. Traditionally, gay communities outside the largest cities have had few formal support organizations and structures other than bars and settings often associated with casual sexual partner-seeking. There have been limited means by which gay men could derive external support for maintaining stable relationships, meet others in social but noncasually sexual ways, and become involved in activities inconsistent with high-risk conduct. It is not likely that the general public will respond to the AIDS crisis by becoming more supportive of social structures in the gay community; to the contrary, homophobic attitudes appear to have increased owing to fear about AIDS. Nonetheless, involvement in organizations of a socially supportive nature, such as service programs for persons with AIDS, gay-affirmative religious organizations, community health and prevention programs, advocacy groups, and social organizations not oriented to casual sexual activities, may embody useful alternatives for individuals seeking to adopt safer life-styles.

Finally, the maintenance of low-risk behavior among both homosexual and heterosexual persons requires a willingness to accept responsibility for the well-being of oneself and others. Research on teenage pregnancy has implicated low self-esteem and low self-pride as determinants of susceptibility to pregnancy; adolescents who become pregnant typically score lower on self-esteem measures than their peers who are either less sexually active or more likely to use effective contraception (Colletta, Gregg, Hadler, Lee, & Mekelburg, 1980; Rosenburg, 1965). In a similar way, susceptibility to serious drug use patterns has been related to poor self-esteem (Kaplan, 1980). While the specific linkages of self-esteem with promiscuity, ability to resist sexual coercion, and resistance to drug use patterns may be indirect, it is logical to assume that AIDS-prevention programs will be most effective when they foster a sense of pride and responsibility for the health of oneself and others. This is, no doubt, equally true regardless of whether the target population is gay men, heterosexuals with multiple partners, adolescents, or persons at risk for intravenous drug use.

Psychosocial Consequences of HIV Seropositivity

Most literature on acquired immune deficiency syndrome (AIDS) has focused on persons with clinical-criterion, or frank, AIDS. Given the lethality of an AIDS diagnosis, the recency of the disease, and the exponential increase in AIDS cases, it is understandable that clinical-criterion AIDS has dominated discussion and research. Relatively less attention has been directed toward those who are HIV-exposed but remain healthy, even though their numbers are substantially greater than the number of persons diagnosed with frank AIDS. This chapter will discuss HIV seropositivity, the reasons that people seek testing, and some of the psychological, behavioral, and social consequences of positive HIV test results. These include voluntary changes in sexual practices, adverse emotional consequences, possible neurological consequences of exposure, and the social consequences of HIV exposure. Chapter 6 will then discuss specific interventions that can assist persons who are adversely affected by the knowledge that they have been exposed to the virus.

5.1. LEARNING OF HIV SEROPOSITIVITY

Individuals learn they have become exposed to the human immunodeficiency virus (HIV) in a variety of ways. Persons who are ill may be tested by their physicians if they have an illness that could be HIV-related and if they are members of an AIDS risk group. Although medical ethics stress the importance of obtaining patients' informed consent before medical procedures are performed (Bayer *et al.*, 1986), some patients may be tested for HIV antibodies as part of a general medical evaluation or during a hospital admission without their prior knowledge or consent. As discussed earlier, testing is now mandatory for persons serving in or entering the military, immigrants seeking entry to the United States, and federal prisoners. Unless specifically prohibited by state law, many insurance companies now require applicants for individual life or health insurance policies to undergo the HIV antibody test before they will be considered insurable. While statutes vary from state to state, other groups, such as marriage license applicants, are required to submit to an HIV test in some areas. Thus, many individuals may be HIV-tested under nonvoluntary circumstances that afford little protection for the privacy or confidentiality of test results.

Since 1985, all blood donations in the United States have been routinely screened for HIV antibodies. While the objective of blood bank screening is to protect blood supplies, blood donors with HIV antibodies may be notified of their positive test result by a telephone call, by mail, or in person if their sample is found to be seropositive. Approximately 55% of persons who donate HIV-infected blood were unaware that they were exposed when they donated the blood (Williams *et al.*, 1987). HIV-positive blood donors who were aware of belonging to an identified risk group but who proceeded to donate blood reported doing so because of peer pressure to donate (29%), specifically to learn their HIV status (29%), or because they believed their blood was a rare type of particular value (61%). Fewer than 6% of antibody-positive blood donors had not taken seriously the appeal for self-deferral by persons in high-risk groups (Williams *et al.*, 1987).

In an effort to discourage use of blood banks to learn the results of an HIV test, all states have developed alternative test sites where HIV antibody testing is available to anyone who voluntarily seeks it.* Laws and

---

*Persons who have any reason to suspect that they could be HIV-infected or who have engaged in AIDS risk activities should never donate blood. In spite of screening, HIV-infected but antibody-negative blood could fail to be detected in the screening process. Alternative HIV test sites were established so that persons could obtain testing at locations other than blood banks. In addition, many blood banks screen samples only with the ELISA test. Given the high probability of false positives with the ELISA, blood banks are a poor site for testing if persons wish to receive accurate information concerning their HIV status.

procedures for reporting positive HIV test results differ from state to state. In some states, individuals are tested anonymously and no identifying information is ever recorded. In other states, the test results and the person's name are reported to state health department officials. One would expect, given the considerable potential for discrimination and stigma associated with seropositivity or AIDS, that those who belong to any of the identified risk groups would be more likely to seek voluntary testing under conditions that afford confidentiality and assure anonymity. There is a need to evaluate whether members of high-risk groups are more likely to utilize programs that provide anonymity relative to those that report test results and identity to health officials.

Several studies have examined the reasons that homosexual men voluntarily seek HIV testing (McKusick, Coates, & Horstman, 1986; Morin, Coates, Woods, & McKusick, 1987). Approximately 39% of gay men who request the test do so specifically to relieve their anxiety about whether they could be HIV-exposed (McKusick, Coates, & Horstman, 1986). Thus, they are hoping for a negative result to reduce anxiety that is already present. This is of concern since an anxious person seeking the reassurance of a negative test result may be ill-prepared to cope with a positive test result. Other reasons for desiring antibody testing are to avoid transmitting the virus to others if exposed (26.7%) or to gain information that will help in planning major life decisions more effectively (10.0%). These latter reasons are consistent with public health recommendations that encourage risk group members to seek voluntary testing in order to increase their motivation to protect both themselves and others from inadvertent infection (U.S. Department of Health and Human Services, 1986a). Persons may also seek voluntary HIV antibody testing to make decisions about pregnancy planning or pregnancy termination because infants born to an HIV-infected mother are themselves often infected. Some individuals prefer to learn their HIV status privately or anonymously before they will be subjected to mandatory testing under less private circumstances, such as military testing or insurance eligibility determinations. If antibody-positive, such individuals can choose to "opt out" of later testing situations that would not afford confidentiality or anonymity.

Most alternative testing sites are reporting dramatic increases in the number of people seeking voluntary testing. However, many of the people who now request the test are at little or no objective risk. This recent influx of minimal- or no-risk test seekers is probably the result of media attention to AIDS and public fears of the disease. The proportion of persons who seek testing and who are genuinely at high risk may actually be decreasing (McKusick, Coates, & Horstman, 1986). Gay men who do not choose to undergo testing report deciding against the test because they believe the results are unclear or lack meaning (32.5%), because they fear breaches in confidentiality (20.9%), or because they fear the anxiety that follows certain knowledge of seropositivity (17.0%) (McKusick, Coates, Horstman, 1986). Other studies find that the anticipation of psychological distress following a positive test result is the single most important reason that risk-group members do not seek testing (Lyter, Valdiserri, Kingsley, Amoroso, & Rinaldo, 1987).

The reasons that persons at risk for AIDS do or do not seek voluntary HIV testing can provide important information for public health AIDS-prevention efforts. Fears of confidentiality breaches and subsequent discrimination, ostracism, or loss of rights if the person's positive antibody status became known represent a significant deterrent to voluntary testing for risk-group members and are not unrealistic concerns. Should public hysteria about AIDS intensify or legislation be be enacted that would deprive HIV-seropositive persons of basic rights and privileges, the populations at greatest risk for HIV infection—particularly gay men and intravenous drug users—may have reason to fear public persecution and unsympathetic discrimination. Guarantees of irrevocable confidentiality and legal protections from any discrimination seem essential if high-risk group members are to be enlisted in voluntary antibody testing efforts.

The assumption that knowledge of one's HIV-antibody status is necessary in order to make risk-behavior change has not been well substantiated. In major cities with well-developed educational campaigns, several large-scale studies show that gay and bisexual men are changing their sexual practices in the direction of reduced risk even without knowing their antibody status (Fox et al., 1987; Johnson & McGrath, 1987; Marlink et al. 1987). Farthing, Jesson, Taylor, Lawrence, and Gazzard (1987) found that 65% of gay men had already modified their sexual behavior before requesting the HIV-antibody test. This suggests that HIV testing, at least for some individuals, is requested after the decision to reduce high-risk conduct has already been made. Other studies demonstrate that HIV test results encourage the continued maintenance of lowered risk activity among persc is who have already reduced their levels of risk behavior (Coates, Morin, & McKusick, 1987; Godfried *et al.*, 1987; Willoughby *et al.*, 1987).

5.2. RISK-BEHAVIOR CHANGES PROMPTED BY SEROPOSITIVITY

Several longitudinal investigations examined changes in the risk behavior of gay men who voluntarily requested HIV-antibody testing and subsequently learned that they were either seropositive or seronegative (Coates, Morin, & McKusick, 1987; Godfried *et al.*, 1987; Joseph *et al.*, 1987; Willoughby *et al.*, 1987). In general, these studies have found that antibody-positive gay men reduced their frequency of high-risk behavior to a greater degree than men who learned they were seronegative. This suggests that for gay and bisexual men, knowledge of seropositivity reinforces efforts to modify risk practices and is consistent with surveys indicating that gay men believe they would be more diligent in maintaining safer sex practices if they learned they were HIV-exposed (Farthing *et al.*, 1987).

While these reported reductions in risk behavior by gay and bisexual men are encouraging, they do not confirm that HIV testing, in and of itself, is sufficient to promote adequate risk-behavior change. Most studies of risk behavior among HIV-seropositive gay males following HIV testing find changes at relative, rather than absolute, levels. For example, in the Willoughby *et al.* (1987) investigation, HIV-exposed persons exhibited greater decreases in the number of different sexual partners (from 9.2 to 5.8) than persons who were seronegative (6.9 to 6.7). However, the clinical and public health significance of these relative changes by HIV-positive persons is unclear. Joseph *et al.* (1987) found that the number of homosexual men who refrained completely from any risk behaviors doubled after persons learned they were seropositive. However, the magnitude of absolute change was small, with an increase from 6.1 to 13.4% of those who refrained from any risk behavior. Similarly, Fox *et al.* (1987) reported that condom use doubled among gay and bisexual men who found they were seropositive but, even so, only one-third of the men were reliably using condoms during anal intercourse.

Several conclusions can be drawn about the effects of knowing one's HIV-exposure status on subsequent risk behavior by gay and bisexual men. First, gay men who learn they are HIV-exposed following voluntary testing make behavior changes in the direction of reduced risk to a greater extent than men who learn they are unexposed. However, the magnitude of change is often modest and may even be less than would occur if the person were engaged in a carefully designed educational or risk-reduction-counseling program regardless of whether or not HIV testing took place (Kelly & St. Lawrence, 1986). As will be discussed in Chapter 6, the type of counseling that follows HIV testing for seropositive persons may also influence the magnitude of behavior change that follows certain knowledge that one has been exposed to the virus.

If the behavior changes made by HIV-positive gay and bisexual men following the test are somewhat encouraging, the relative lack of behavior change among persons who find they are seronegative after testing is cause for discouragement. The same studies that have shown relative decreases in high-risk behavior after notification of seropositivity show little differential risk-behavior change for those who find they are seronegative. Instead of motivating persons to diligently adopt reduced-risk behavior and preserve their unexposed status, negative antibody test result feedback may lead some individuals to believe they are "protected" from AIDS and to continue risky practices. Effective counseling strategies for persons who learn they are seronegative are also needed.

Most of the studies evaluating the effects of HIV testing on subsequent risk behavior have examined seropositive gay and bisexual men. These studies consistently show that about 75% of gay and bisexual men have attempted to change their behavior by reducing the number of sexual partners and sexual practices that allow viral transmission (Johnson & McGrath, 1987; Joseph et al., 1987; McKusick et al., 1987; Nyanjom et al., 1987). One of the factors that predict safe sex adherence by homosexual men is age. Men over 30 are more likely to alter their behavior in the direction of greater safety than are younger men (Schechter et al., 1987). In addition, sexual behavior between partners in a stable relationship is less likely than sexual behavior between casual partners to consistently adhere to safe sex guidelines (McKusick et al., 1987). The belief that one is capable of making the recommended changes to safe sexual practices is the single most powerful predictor of successful risk reduction (McKusick et al., 1987).

Intravenous drug users and heterosexuals with multiple sexual partners have made fewer spontaneous changes in their sexual behavior than gay and bisexual men (Alter, Francis, *et al.*, 1987; Flynn, Jain, *et al.*, 1987; Kegels, Catania, & Coates, 1987; Marlink *et al.*, 1987). In one study, approximately 75% of intravenous drug users continued sharing contaminated needles and engaging in sexual practices that posed transmission risk even following an educational intervention (Flynn, Jain, *et al.*, 1987). Relatively little is known about the effects of HIV-antibody test results on intravenous drug users or heterosexuals with multiple partners. Clearly, this is an area in need of further investigation. In addition, there may be differences in the risk-behavior change of persons who learn they are seropositive following voluntary, as opposed to mandatory, testing. Further research is also needed to address these questions.

5.3. EMOTIONAL CONSEQUENCES THAT FOLLOW KNOWLEDGE OF SEROPOSITIVITY

Learning that one has been exposed to the human immunodeficiency virus almost invariably precipitates emotional distress for the individual, as well as for sexual partners, friends, and family who are aware of the individual's exposure status (Joseph *et al.*, 1987; Pollak, Gharakhanian, Rozenbaum, Viallefont, & Aine, 1987). Even if asymptomatic and without any symptoms of clinical illness, the person may have to cope with years of uncertainty about future health. It is not yet possible to predict with certainty the long-term health consequences of HIV infection on an individual basis, so the HIV-seropositive person lives with the constant fear of developing AIDS. Knowledge of seropositivity typically produces elevations on measures of psychological distress that are 2 to 3 standard deviations above the norms for a general population and similar to the norms for psychiatric outpatients (Jacobson, Perry, Scavuzzo, & Roberts, 1987). The most common psychological reactions to HIV seropositivity are anxiety, anger, depression, somatization, and denial (Coates, Morin, & McKusick, 1987; McCusker *et al.*, 1987; Miller *et al.*, 1987).

5.3.1. Anxiety

Predictably, anxiety is one of the most common reactions to HIV seropositivity (Coates, Morin, & McKusick, 1987). More than 50% of test-positive homosexual men report experiencing significant anxiety, insomnia, and memory problems after learning they are HIV-exposed (Joseph *et al.,* 1987; Pollak, Gharakhanian, *et al.,* 1987). Others have reported that reactive adjustment disorders reflecting increased stress and anxiety are observed in 75% of those infected with HIV (Tross, Hirsch, Babkin, Berry, & Holland, 1987). Some fears are general, while others are highly specific. General fears revolve around the fear of developing AIDS, the stress of coping with ambiguity about future health and loss of control at the prospect of a future orchestrated by an unobservable virus.

Specific fears include fear of becoming ill, anticipation of future pain or disfigurement, and concern over the possible loss of social or relationship supports. The latter fears are sometimes realistic, for disclosure of HIV seropositivity can result in increasing distance between the HIV-exposed person and those social supports that had been available before the person learned of seropositivity. In its most extreme form, the person anticipates abandonment by everyone who has previously been part of his or her social network. Other common fears revolve around the possibility of future helplessness or dependency. This feared dependency may be physical or financial as the person imagines future scenarios involving loss of employment with its attendant loss of income and eventual depletion of savings. Anxiety may be even more intense for the homosexual persons whose life-style is not generally known to family, friends, or co-workers owing to expectations of censure and rejection if HIV status and sexual preference become simultaneously known to others.

5.3.2. Anger

Homosexual men who are seropositive experience significantly higher levels of anger than men who are seronegative or who do not know their HIV status (McCusker *et al.,* 1987). Anger can result from the feared progression from HIV infection to AIDS, the social discrimination and stigmatization encountered by HIV-affected persons, the lack of effective treatments to eliminate the virus, and the absence of any reassurance that medical solutions will emerge in the near future. Persons struggling to come to grips with their own seropositivity can be further angered by the callous, indifferent, or hostile reactions they may encounter. Thoughtless casual comments by others who are unaware of the person's infection status or tasteless jokes about AIDS impact with highly personal meaning upon the person newly aware of HIV exposure. HIV-seropositive gay men may become angered and hostile at the indifference that they hear others express concerning AIDS. For example, some fundamentalists have described AIDS as "God's retribution for the sin of homosexuality," an attribution that implies the affected person is deserving of disease and death. Self-directed anger is also common, including anger over past behavior, anger toward persons who may have exposed them, and anger over the failure to make behavior change in time to prevent exposure. Because AIDS is widely perceived as a disease associated with homosexuality, persons with HIV infection who are hemophiliacs, transfusion recipients, or heterosexuals may be particularly angry and frustrated concerning their status. Recent media reports of protests and demonstrations reflect the anger felt by HIV-exposed persons, as well as by those with more advanced stages of HIV illness.

Occasionally, anger is manifested in maladaptive coping attempts, such as excessive drinking or drug abuse, following news of HIV exposure. Such substance overuse may reflect anger; at other times it represents a maladaptive escape from psychological distress. This is of special concern because excessive alcohol intake and some recreational drugs have immunosuppressant effects that may interact with HIV infection to further compromise the person's future health. In addition, because intoxicants are behavioral disinhibitors, the person may engage in impulsive behavior that would not occur otherwise.

5.3.3. Depression

Levels of depression are significantly higher among persons who have tested positive for the virus than for those who are seronegative or unaware of their antibody status (Coates, Morin, & McKusick, 1987; Cochran, 1987; McCusker *et al.*, 1987). Approximately 50% of test-positive individuals experience reactive depression (Joseph *et al.*, 1987; Pollak, Gharakhanian, *et al.*, 1987), often in the range of clinical depression (Eisdorfer, 1987a).

Ruminations and obsessional thinking are common in persons who recently learned of their HIV exposure. Common obsessive thoughts revolve around themes of contamination, guilt, and the unfairness of their situation. Guilt may especially focus on past behavior and life-style, or about the possibility of having transmitted the virus to others. Sadness, hopelessness, withdrawal, isolation, lethargy, and other symptoms of depression are often present. It is not unusual to encounter individuals who respond to their HIV seropositivity by quitting their jobs, disposing of their goods and property, and awaiting the AIDS death they fear. Thoughts of suicide are common among HIV-exposed individuals (Eisdorfer, 1987a). The onset of depressive symptoms may also mask the early signs of neurological involvement, making differential diagnosis difficult (Eisdorfer, 1987a).

5.3.4. Somatization

Persons who are seropositive consistently report higher levels of psychosomatic distress and more physical symptoms than men who are seronegative or who are unaware of their HIV status. Some of the common complaints are consistent with early symptoms of ARC or AIDS, but many are not, reflecting the individual's misinterpretation of common physical sensations. Cochran (1987) found that one-third of the symptom complaints of healthy but seropositive persons were actually inconsistent with an ARC or AIDS diagnosis. Thus, many of the subjective symptoms detected by HIV-positive persons reflect preoccupation with illness rather than actual physical changes.

Fear of AIDS has made gay men, in particular, highly vigilant of symptoms that might not have been noticed in the past. Spots and blemishes, aches and pains, or minor fatigue become cause for alarm that AIDS is developing. These problems are exacerbated for those who know they are HIV-positive. Realistic concern about one's health is reasonable and a common outcome of seropositivity, but it may alternate with exaggerated sensitivity and somatic preoccupation.

5.3.5. Denial

Denial of HIV infection is of particular concern since recent evidence suggests that denial is the single strongest predictor of failure to take risk-reduction steps (Joseph et al., 1987). A consistent pattern of findings indicates that although most HIV-infected persons make behavior changes in the direction of reduced risk and responsible conduct, not everyone responds to seropositivity with increased safety or behavior change (Joseph et al., 1987; Nyanjom et al., 1987; Stempel, Moulton, Kelly, Osmond, & Moss, 1987; Stevens, Taylor, Zang, Rodriguez de Cordoba, & Rubenstein, 1987). Denial may be self-protective in the short term because it reduces emotional distress (Douglas, Harper, & Polk, 1987). The long-term danger, however, is that denial precludes making the behavioral changes that will prevent further HIV transmission or repeated exposure to the virus.

Intravenous drug users evidence considerably higher levels of denial than homosexual or bisexual men. Even with individual long-term counseling, medical follow-up, and the opportunity for methadone maintenance, 67% of HIV-seropositive drug users revert to drug use within 6 months, as compared with 7% for the entire population of drug users and to 24% of seronegative users in one established methadone maintenance program over the same period (Marlink *et al.*, 1987). This population is of concern since continued needle sharing in combination with unchanged sexual behavior carries high potential for transmission of HIV infection to others. Other research found that even when intravenous drug users were knowledgeable about HIV transmission and had disinfecting solutions readily available in the setting where they used and shared drug paraphernalia, 77% continued sharing their drug paraphernalia and very rarely disinfected needles between uses (Flynn, Jain, *et al.*, 1987).

Not surprisingly, denial of the personal threat from AIDS is also more evident among the young. Younger men report less effort to change their sexual behavior. For example, one study found that 68% of gay men over 40 reduced risk behavior even before HIV testing, while only 49% of the men under 30 had made such risk-behavior change prior to learning their HIV status (Schechter *et al.*, 1987). Younger persons are also more reluctant to learn whether they have become HIV-exposed and are less likely to seek HIV testing (McCusker *et al.*, 1987).

5.4. NEUROLOGICAL CONSEQUENCES OF HIV EXPOSURE

There is now strong evidence that HIV is neurotropic and can infect the central nervous system within a very short time after exposure to the virus (Wolcott, 1986b). Cerebrospinal fluid (CSF) abnormalities are common in HIV-infected persons, even those without any overt neuropsychiatric symptoms. Approximately 43% of asymptomatic but HIV-positive gay men evidence measurable CSF abnormalities (Collier, Coombs, Nikora, Corey, & Handsfield, 1987; McArthur *et al.*, 1987). The clinical significance of HIV in cerebrospinal fluid is unclear and has not been consistently linked to identifiable neurological deficits (Collier, Coombs, *et al.*, 1987; Katlana, Rey, Salmon, Ngovan, & Dazza, 1987; McArthur *et al.*, 1987). However, in one study (Janssen *et al.*, 1987), 50% of the seropositive persons evidenced some neurological abnormality compared with only 8% of the seronegative controls. Most of the impairment was mild, suggesting that subtle neurological manifestations may be common following HIV exposure but are not clinically evident in most HIV-exposed persons.

Ten percent of those who eventually develop ARC or AIDS will have some neurological impairment as the *first* indication of their future illness (Wolcott, 1986b). These initial neurological cues may precede any further clinical signs of ARC or AIDS by as much as 12 months (Levy, Bredesen, & Rosenblum, 1985). Aseptic meningitis and herpes zoster radiculitis are the most common presenting neurological syndromes, often presaging the later development of ARC and AIDS (Wolcott, 1986b).

5.5. SOCIAL CONSEQUENCES OF HIV INFECTION

The social disruptions that often follow HIV infection are twofold. Some are by-products from the emotional upset of the person who learns of certain HIV exposure. Other social difficulties stem from avoidance or fear of others, which increases the person's sense of isolation. Anxiety, depression, and anger are often detrimental to interpersonal relationships. In addition, HIV-positive persons may withdraw from social contact. Pollack, Gharakhanian, *et al.* (1987) found that most HIV-positive persons spent more time in solitary activities after they learned they were seropositive, and most feared that their HIV exposure would negatively affect established relationships. More than half of those who were in steady relationships hesitated to inform their partner, fearing they would precipitate a breakup in the relationship. There is some evidence to suggest that such fears may be realistic. HIV seropositivity led to dissolution of existing relationships for approximately one-third of the couples Pollak, Gharakhanian, *et al.* (1987) surveyed, and couple disruption was equally common among heterosexual and homosexual couples. Other researchers have also found that relationships were more likely to end after one partner learned of seropositivity (Coates, Morin, & McKusick, 1987).

Social isolation is not necessarily the inevitable outcome from positive HIV test results. In San Francisco, a survey found that gay men who disclosed their positive antibody status to others reported disclosure to be either helpful, or neither helpful nor harmful (Zones, Beeson, Echenberg, Rutherford, & O'Malley, 1987). However, the results from San Francisco differ from findings reported from other areas and are probably a function of the relatively supportive social environment for gay men in the San Francisco area. Thus, in an affirmative environment, test disclosure can be constructive and serve as a means for generating social support.

Avoidant reactions of others can unwittingly heighten distress and leave the HIV-positive person feeling shunned, vulnerable, and isolated from the very persons who had previously been a dependable support group. Because learning of HIV exposure often produces an emotional crisis, strong social supports are especially needed during this time. A strong network of family and friends can be important in helping the person to cope with this adjustment. Unfortunately, many homosexuals and drug users are estranged from their families, are already negatively stigmatized by society, and may lack other social supports. Some persons retreat into a self-imposed isolation, fearing reexposure to new infections, out of concern over transmitting the virus to others, or simply because they are stunned by the news of their exposure. Obsessional thinking hinders both concentration and responsivity to others, leaving many persons unable to maintain their usual investment in work or close personal relationships to the same extent as before learning of their seropositivity. During a personal crisis, it is common for people to become more self-absorbed and less sensitive to others. This is no less true during the personal crisis that often follows learning of HIV exposure. The meaning that an infected person attaches to seropositivity may also contribute to social isolation. Self-labeling oneself as "diseased," "infected," or "contaminated" can foster self-isolation and feelings that the HIV-affected person no longer belongs in the mainstream.

When seropositivity becomes known, there may be a loss of relationships and social supports, and even people who desire to maintain their social support systems may discover that others are now fearful and avoidant of them. Thus, even when the HIV-exposed person responds to seropositivity in emotionally healthy ways, the reactions of others can produce social isolation and rejection.

5.6. IMPLICATIONS FOR FUTURE HEALTH AND ADJUSTMENT

Virtually all research has found that significant emotional and social distress follow learning of exposure to human immunodeficiency virus. While the studies in this area have usually examined the reactions of gay and bisexual men, there is no reason to believe that others react any differently or experience less emotional distress. The psychological and social support needs of the hundreds of thousands of persons who will eventually learn, following HIV testing, that they are HIV-antibody-positive are among the least recognized and most insufficiently addressed mental health aspects of the present health crisis.

Closer attention is warranted to the psychological consequences of HIV seropositivity for several reasons. Clearly, one reason is to provide interventions that can alleviate, to the greatest degree possible, the emotional and social distress that often follows notification that one is HIV-infected. Additionally, persons who are able to cope effectively with the anxiety engendered by seropositivity may be better able to implement the behavior changes that will protect others from infection and themselves from possible viral reexposure. Maladaptive responses such as denial or intoxicant overuse no doubt predict poor long-term adherence to risk-reduction recommendations. To the extent that healthy but HIV-positive individuals can accept the implications of their infection status on future sexual conduct and can channel their anxiety in constructive directions, they may be better able to implement behavioral changes that will also protect themselves and others.

Although it is not yet well substantiated, there is the possibility that maladaptive coping behavior by HIV-infected persons could directly influence their future health course, since high stress levels can have immunosuppressant effects of their own (Antoni, 1987; Coates, Temoshok, & Mandel, 1984; Penzien, 1986). Psychoimmunology research examining the effect of psychological stress on disease susceptibility has found that an active, instrumental coping style produces greater differences in both physiology and behavior than a passive, helpless reaction (Antoni, 1987). The passive, helpless coping style is of particular concern since it is associated with corticosteroid elevations, suppression of the immune system, and depression (Antoni, 1987; Selye, 1946, 1956), and because elevated levels of corticosteroids produce suppression in T lymphocytes (Antoni, 1987; Cupps & Fauci, 1982; Felton, Carolson, Olschowka, & Livnat, 1985). Thus, it is possible that the way in which a person copes with stress may differentially affect subsequent immune functioning. Transient stressors are of less concern than prolonged stress, for it is the enduring stressors that produce measurable changes in immune system functioning (Antoni, 1987). Other viral diseases that are immune-mediated, such as recurrent herpes labialis, are exacerbated by stress (Luborsky, Mintz, Brightman, & Katcher, 1976). The possibility that emotional coping could influence future health after HIV exposure is also reason to more closely address the psychological needs of those who become HIV-seropositive.

Psychosocial Interventions
for HIV-Seropositive Persons

Asymptomatic but HIV-seropositive persons are the largest group of individuals affected by AIDS. Some HIV-infected persons may live for the rest of their lives without developing physical symptoms but remain capable of transmitting the virus. Some will develop physical symptoms and future health compromises, while others will progress to frank AIDS. Without doubt, knowledge of one's own seropositivity precipitates a host of questions, uncertainties, and health anxieties for which there are few reassurances. Several million Americans are already infected with the human immunodeficiency virus and, despite the well-documented and detrimental psychological consequences of HIV infection, little clinical research has yet appeared to guide the mental health professionals who will soon be seeing the growing number of HIV-exposed persons.

There are several reasons why mental health professionals have not always perceived significant roles for themselves in the AIDS health crisis (Coates *et al.*, 1984). Since viral diseases are not the usual subject matter of psychology, counseling, social work, or other helping areas, professionals in these areas may regard AIDS-related conditions as the exclusive province of biological medicine. Yet, as we have already seen, no biomedical preventions for AIDS are available now, and medical treatments for AIDS are highly limited. Assisting persons who experience emotional upset following notification of seropositivity is in the province of mental health practitioners. In addition, persons who are HIV-exposed may require assistance to discontinue practices that can transmit the virus to others or can expose themselves to further reinfection. Even for those who know they are HIV-seropositive, making risk-reduction behavioral changes is difficult and may require assistance as new self-management skills are being learned to replace risky past behavior patterns. Clinicians may also believe they have no role in the treatment of a terminal diagnosis, unaware that many individuals have stages of HIV infection with less ominous outcomes than frank AIDS and are in need of mental health services.

In this chapter, interventions for HIV-affected persons will be described. Although the reactive emotional distress that often follows HIV seropositivity has been well documented, the literature evaluating specific interventions to ameliorate distress among HIV-affected persons is less developed. However, substantial information regarding effective interventions with other populations who experience similar emotional distress patterns can be extended to HIV-seropositive persons. Case examples will illustrate how these intervention methods can be applied in therapy with HIV-exposed persons. Because a detailed guide to therapy techniques is beyond the scope of this book, readers unfamiliar with the clinical procedures described in this chapter may wish to consult the specialized resources to which references are made.

6.1. COUNSELING AT THE TIME OF HIV TESTING

It is essential to ensure that persons who seek testing understand the meaning of an HIV test and receive counseling to help cope with the test results. While this seems logical and straightforward, one large-scale study (McKusick, Coates, & Horstman, 1986) found that only 59% of the individuals who completed HIV testing received any precounseling about the test or the meaning of its results, and only 50% of those who had the test received their test results face to face. The balance learned of their HIV test results by telephone or mail, with little or no feedback about the test's interpretation. Others may receive test result feedback face to face, but from a staff member who is uncomfortable providing the information or discussing it. When test results are conveyed by a staff member who states the result bluntly and, in some cases, reads information from a standard counseling brochure, the client is unlikely to inquire more fully about the test results, about their interpretation, or about future courses of action. It is also quite common for an HIV test result to be misunderstood. One common misconception is that HIV seropositivity is equivalent to an AIDS diagnosis. Frequently, HIV-seropositive persons are so numbed by the anxiety of a positive test result that it may take several days before questions arise. When referral resources are not provided with the test results, the individual may not know where to turn for reliable information. McKusick, Coates, and Horstman (1986) found that fewer than 33% of test recipients received any referral information after being advised they were HIV-positive, despite substantial evidence that learning of HIV exposure is highly stressful. The authors are aware of occasions when the information that is provided after HIV testing is inaccurate or reflects insensitive biases unsupported by the literature. For example, one patient who asked his physician what to do after receiving a positive result reported to us being told to "become heterosexual."

The need for adequate pre- and posttest counseling is not limited to HIV-seropositive persons alone; those receiving a negative result should also be counseled. A negative antibody result can be detrimental if the person feels false security based on the result. If seronegativity is interpreted as a reassuring license to delay changing the risk practices that prompted interest in testing in the first place, then the negative result could actually perpetuate continued high risk. Finally, and as discussed earlier, a single negative result cannot be interpreted as clear evidence that the person is free of HIV infection because detectable antibodies may not appear for months following viral exposure. During that time, the person may be infected but still test negative for HIV antibodies (Polis *et al.*, 1987). Therefore, information, counseling, and education should be provided even for those who are seronegative.

For all of these reasons, counseling before and counseling after testing are both essential. Gold, Seymour, and Sahl (1986) have described a model voluntary and anonymous HIV testing program in California that incorporates many useful elements. The availability of the HIV test is advertised and disseminated widely, including in the newspapers. Persons interested in learning more about the test may telephone a hot line and receive information to help them decide whether to pursue testing further. If they wish to proceed with HIV testing, an appointment is scheduled over the telephone. Names are not requested at any point.

Instead, the callers are asked to devise an identification code and to subsequently use the self-devised code instead of a name.

6.1.1. Pretest Counseling and Education

All persons receive precounseling when they first arrive at a test site and before the test is ever administered. Upon arriving at the program described by Gold *et al.* (1986), each person views a 10-minute videotape that describes the test in detail. Following the film, a staff counselor leads a small group discussion in which people are asked to think about the difference between *assuming* they are HIV-positive and *knowing* that they are seropositive. Persons willing to assume that they are HIV-positive because of past risk behavior may not need the test if they are willing to make the necessary behavioral changes without the trauma of a positive result (Gold *et al.*, 1986). On the other hand, those who delay changing their risk behavior may be propelled into action by a positive test result. During group discussion, questions are encouraged and persons who have sensitive questions can meet individually with a counselor who provides assistance in reaching a decision about whether to proceed with HIV testing.

As discussed in Chapter 5, several studies have found that the reasons people request HIV testing are often psychological (McKusick, Coates, & Horstman, 1986; Morin *et al.*, 1987). Approximately 39% request the test hoping for reassurance that they are unexposed (McKusick, Coates, & Horstman, 1986). If the results do not confirm that desired outcome, these individuals may be ill-equipped to deal with the certainty of their HIV exposure. Therefore, the precounseling session might usefully include an assessment of whether test seekers are prepared to cope with a positive HIV result. The addition of role-playing or behavior rehearsal to the pretest counseling session may prove helpful in this regard. The counselor can role-play giving both a negative and a positive result, and the counselor and the client together can explore whether the person is truly prepared for either result and ready to proceed with testing, or whether testing should be deferred.

In the program described by Gold *et al.* (1986), those who decide to proceed with HIV testing have blood samples drawn after counseling and receive an appointment to return 2 weeks later. Since the 2-week waiting interval can be a difficult time, participants are provided with a list of available resources for use during the waiting period if needed.

6.1.2. Posttest Counseling

Upon returning 2 weeks later, each client meets individually with a counselor to receive the test result. Blood samples initially positive with the ELISA screening are confirmed with the Western blot test before results are conveyed. The meaning of the test result is explained and clarified, and community referrals are provided. The interview also addresses substance use, the individual's emotional reaction to the test result, and how to inform others of the test result. A "follow-up" videotape is shown and the person receives a resource list of mental health professionals before leaving the test site. The goals of the posttest session are threefold: (1) to help the person absorb the news and cope with the results, (2) to provide the person with available resources, and (3) to counsel as much as possible about health education, risk reduction, and safer sex (Gold *et al.*, 1986).

Since people are often numb following a positive result, they may experience a delayed emotional reaction after leaving the office. For this reason, each person leaves with the referral list and a specific referral to an area counselor. Common issues that arise during the posttest session include substance abuse, fear of sex, relationship conflicts, grief over anticipated losses, health concerns, anxiety, how to tell and whom to tell, quality-of-life issues, how to change sexual behavior, health planning, and fear of illness (Gold *et al.*, 1986). Other issues, such as whether to disclose homosexual preference or drug use to others, may also arise and require attention during the posttest counseling session.

6.2. PSYCHOSOCIAL INTERVENTIONS TO PROMOTE BEHAVIOR CHANGE AND COPING SKILLS

The sections that follow present intervention strategies that can be helpful when working with HIV-seropositive persons. Some of these interventions reduce the emotional distress that often follows HIV seropositivity, while others assist the person in changing risk behavior. Although HIV-positive clients may be seen in individual therapy, group interventions can be particularly helpful because they create social supports within the group, reduce the social isolation that often follows HIV seropositivity, and enable the client to realize that others are coping with the same adjustment. As constructive coping efforts are described by other group members, the HIV-positive client can benefit from their experiences and solutions.

6.2.1. Interventions to Alter Continued Risk Behavior

All of the interventions described in Chapter 3 for prevention are also applicable with HIV-seropositive individuals or groups. The interventions remain the same, although the focus shifts from preventing exposure to protecting others by not engaging in behavior that can transmit HIV and to protecting oneself from possible reexposure. Information provision and education about risk practices provide the client with an accurate informational base and counter various misconceptions. Assistance in making the transition from high-risk sexual activities is as important for persons who know they are HIV-seropositive as it is for clients who are simply worried and at risk for AIDS. Interventions may include self-management training to identify factors that led to past high-risk behavior and to develop specific behavioral strategies for dealing with those situations in new and more adaptive ways. Assertion training may be warranted to help the person learn to refuse coercive sexual overtures skillfully and comfortably. If the seropositive client is an intravenous drug user, education, self-management, and assertion training should target not only risky sexual practices but also drug use behavior. All of the intervention components discussed in Chapter 3 are also relevant to the treatment of persons who know they are HIV-seropositive.

Some persons respond to their seropositivity with fear of further sexual intimacy and choose to become abstinent. For some, abstinence is a lasting life-style choice, but for others, it may be a transient reaction. Even when individuals report they intend to become celibate, information about safer sexual practices should still be provided. If the person should resume sexual activity, the likelihood of engaging in activities that permit HIV transmission will be reduced. Thus, risk-reduction interventions for an HIV-seropositive person who is not sexually active are prophylactic and anticipate the possibility that sexual activity may occur at some time in the future. In order to protect the health and rights of others, clients who know they are seropositive should be counseled that it is ethical and responsible to inform potential sexual partners of their HIV-antibody status (U.S. Department of Health and Human Services, 1986b).

HIV-seropositive persons can also be assisted to make behavior changes to promote their general fitness and well-being. Although there is not yet firm evidence that proper diet, nutrition, regular sleep, or exercise impacts on the health course of those with HIV infection, persons with other diseases benefit from such healthful regimens. A study of long-term survivors of frank AIDS has reported a tentative relationship between physical exercise and long-term survival (Temoshok, Zich, Solomon, & Stites, 1987), and sound nutrition, fitness, and healthful regimens may influence susceptibility to illness. Even in the absence of clear empirical support to date, few clinicians would argue against increasing health-promotion strategies for any client, especially when they cannot be to the client's detriment and may have positive benefit. Another advantage from this aspect of treatment is that it provides HIV-affected persons with a concrete and constructive course for positive action focused on living fully, rather than on the prospect of future illness. Many clients find that when they engage in specific behavior-change steps to enhance their health and fitness, a sense of personal control is restored.

In addition to promoting healthful life-style changes, it is prudent for the therapist to evaluate whether the client is engaging in practices that could worsen health. Chronic overuse of common recreational drugs such as alcohol or marijuana have independent immunosuppressive properties (Goedert, 1985). Given their higher risk of immune system compromise, it is wise to counsel HIV-infected persons to eliminate practices that could negatively influence future health, including alcohol overuse, marijuana or cigarette smoking, and the use of other chemical substances such as inhaled nitrites. Intoxicating substances are of particular concern because they are behavioral disinhibitors that can contribute to risky sexual behavior patterns that would not otherwise occur. Should the client be chemically dependent, substance use interventions are warranted, or the client may require referral to a more specialized substance use treatment program.

6.2.2. Psychological Interventions to Reduce Stress Associated with Seropositivity

Although anxiety is one of the most common reactions to HIV seropositivity, anxiety is not necessarily detrimental. It can be helpful when it becomes the impetus for making behavior changes to reduce future reexposure risk, to discontinue practices that would permit viral transmission, and to adopt more healthful styles of living. However, anxiety levels are detrimental when they interfere with the client's comfort and effectiveness in daily life and create subjective misery. Excessive anxiety may also contribute to a sense of helplessness in which the person feels little control over the present or the future and continues maladaptive behavior patterns.

Anxiety reduction is an important psychosocial intervention strategy for helping asymptomatic or minimally symptomatic HIV-exposed persons to acquire effective coping skills and to overcome preoccupations that impair their daily functioning. Therapists walk a delicate line in implementing anxiety-reduction strategies because there is no reassurance that the feared progression to AIDS will not occur. For some clients, that feared future will eventually become reality. When using anxiety-reduction procedures, therapists can emphasize that the development of AIDS is not a present reality, and, while no one can promise that it will not happen, incapacitating fears compromise the client's current quality of life. The therapist can suggest that if the person's future health changes, then those changes can be addressed as they occur. HIV-seropositive clients' fear of AIDS has some basis in reality, and it is unjustified to pretend otherwise.

In any form of therapy intervention, it is essential that the therapist develop rapport and a sensitive, accurate understanding of the client's feelings, distress, and current coping style. For HIV-seropositive clients whose daily functioning is compromised by anxiety, specific attention may need to be directed toward anxiety symptoms. Because anxiety entails physiological, cognitive, and behavioral components, therapists may choose to intervene in any of these areas. However, one of the most widely used and well-researched clinical strategies for helping clients cope with anxiety is relaxation training.

Relaxation training is intended to provide the client with a skill that can be used to counter feelings of maladaptive, debilitating anxiety. A number of relaxation procedures are available to therapists. Progressive deep muscle relaxation, originally introduced by Jacobson (1938), is one of the most frequently used procedures. During a 20- to 30-minute progressive relaxation exercise, the client's attention is directed toward the sensations that are produced when various muscle groups are tensed and then relaxed. Each muscle group receives individual attention as the therapist verbally instructs the client to successively tense and relax muscles in all body areas. Jacobson recognized that for the technique to have therapeutic value, it must be extended into the person's daily life. As a result, clients are also usually trained to practice the relaxation exercise each day and to develop the habit of relaxing throughout the day those muscles that are not in use, a procedure called "differential relaxation." For example, a person sitting at a desk might be taught to relax the shoulders, torso, and lower body while talking on the telephone, thus differentially relaxing the muscles that are not in active use. The person may be instructed to relax muscles in the arms and legs while talking, or the facial muscles while driving a car. With practice, the procedures produce emotional calming effects. An excellent guide to progressive relaxation training techniques can be found in Goldfried and Davison's (1976) text on behavior therapy. Deep muscle relaxation can also be achieved with hypnosis, transcendental meditation, or autogenic training, although these procedures may take longer to become effective than behavioral training methods.

Cue-controlled relaxation is a variation of relaxation training in which the person learns to relax in response to a thought word or "cue" (Cautela, 1966; Grimm, 1980). Cue-controlled relaxation is usually taught after progressive muscle relaxation training and is practiced over several therapy sessions. After deep muscle relaxation has been induced, the therapist pairs relaxation with a cue word such as *relax* or *calm*. The client may be instructed to focus on slow, regular breathing while in a relaxed state and to think of the word *relax* (or a similar cue word) each time he or she exhales. The therapist vocalizes the cue word for several exhalations and then has the person continue to practice thinking the cue word with each exhalation. Following a number of such pairings, the person is instructed to remain relaxed. After a pause of several minutes, the cue word procedure is repeated. Over time, and as a result of the association between relaxation and the cue word, clients become better able to relax themselves by focusing on relaxed breathing and repeating the cue word. Typically, the person is instructed to apply cue-controlled relaxation at the first signs of anxiety or tension in day-to-day living.

Relaxing imagery has also been used as an adjunct to relaxation training. In this variation, the client is asked to recall a particularly relaxing and pleasant memory from the past, and to describe the image in detail to the therapist. At the conclusion of a relaxation training exercise and when relaxation has been induced, the therapist describes the visual image and asks the client to imagine that image. Over therapy sessions, the progressive muscle instructions are abbreviated and the patient is instructed to recreate the visual image when anxiety is present and to respond to the visual imagery with relaxation.

Relaxation training may be used alone or in combination with other interventions and is a component in broad-spectrum stress management interventions (Meichenbaum, 1975; Meichenbaum & Jaremko, 1983). Since uncontrolled stress produces transient impairments in immune system functioning (Kiecolt-Glaser & Glaser, 1987) and because such stress-related immunosuppression may have important consequences for HIV-exposed persons, stress management training may be seen as a potential prophylactic for HIV-exposed persons and for addressing symptoms of anxiety and tension. While relaxation training usually takes place in a therapy session, clients are usually given tape recordings of the therapist's exercise instructions and are asked also to practice relaxing with the tape at home between visits. As a client becomes proficient in the skill of self-relaxation, the therapist and the client together identify stressful events, thoughts, or situations that have instigated maladaptive anxiety. The client is then instructed and guided in applying anxiety management and self-relaxation efforts at those times (cf. Swinn, 1977, 1980; Swinn & Deffenbacher, 1982).

Clinical research literature documents the usefulness of relaxation training with a variety of health-related conditions. Relaxation training significantly alleviates anxiety and reduces treatment side effects in cancer patients (Burish, Carey, Krozely, & Greco, 1987; Lyles, Burish, Krozely, & Oldham, 1982; Morrow, 1984), reduces postpartum distress (Halonen & Passman, 1985), and has proven effective in the treatment of essential hypertension (Hoelscher, Lichstein, Fischer, & Hegarty, 1987), headache (Andrasik, Blanchard, Neff, & Rodichok, 1984), and other forms of pain management (Funch & Gale, 1984). Relaxation training and education improves the physical, psychological, and life-style status of patients who survive myocardial infarctions, and measurable improvements are sustained even 12 months following their hospital discharge (Oldenburg, Perkins, & Andrews, 1985). A substantial body of literature affirms that relaxation training lowers both the experience of anxiety and the physical discomforts associated with sustained anxiety.

Stress management training, which usually employs both relaxation therapy and techniques to assist the client in changing stressful cognitive patterns, has been especially effective for treating illnesses with symptoms that are exacerbated by anxiety. When such a multicomponent anxiety management program was implemented for the treatment of irritable bowel syndrome, patients improved and the benefits from stress management training were maintained through a 2-year follow-up (Neff

& Blanchard, 1987). A few studies have specifically evaluated the usefulness of stress management training with persons who have sexually transmitted diseases. When stress management training was compared with traditional psychoanalytic therapy or a self-help condition for persons with genital herpes (Drob, Bernard, Lifshutz, & Nierenberg, 1986), the behavioral stress management treatment produced significantly more improvement in anxiety levels, depression, affect, communication, sexuality, self-confidence, and interpersonal relationships than did the other two interventions.

One study has specifically evaluated the efficacy of stress management intervention for persons who are HIV-seropositive (Coates & McKusick, 1987). In this study, 60 antibody-positive persons who had lymphadenopathy but were otherwise healthy were randomly assigned to stress management training or a waiting list control condition. The 8-week stress management program included relaxation training, cognitive coping strategies, and intervention to improve relationship skills and health habits. At the conclusion of the intervention, participants in the stress management groups displayed significantly less stress and depression, lower rates of high-risk sexual behavior capable of transmitting HIV, and better immune functioning than persons in the control condition. Thus, stress reduction may be of particular benefit when counseling HIV-seropositive persons.

The following case example illustrates how a relaxation training intervention can be implemented with a seropositive client.

6.2.2.1. Case Example

The client, a 26-year-old female with a history of intravenous drug use and multiple heterosexual contacts with male drug users 5 years earlier, was referred for therapy several months after learning she was HIV-seropositive. An HIV-antibody test was performed when the client sought medical assistance at a clinic during a bout of influenza and told the clinic physician that she had been an intravenous drug user in the past and was frightened of AIDS. Feedback about her positive antibody test result was provided during a return visit to the health clinic, although the client was unable to recall the specific information she was given at the time about the test result or its meaning. The client was not drug-dependent at the time she sought therapy, and although she was

HIV-seropositive, she had no clear clinical evidence of HIV illness.

The client requested therapy to deal with anxiety symptoms, including tension headaches, restlessness, nightmares, sleep-onset insomnia, an inability to concentrate, and worry over her future health. She reported using alcohol and smoking marijuana, sometimes at high levels, in an effort to alleviate her anxiety and worry. Although employed, the client was concerned that she would lose her job as a result of anxiety and the maladaptive ways she was attempting to cope with her distress.

Because it was unclear whether the client understood the meaning of HIV seropositivity or the difference between asymptomatic infection and AIDS, these informational issues were discussed in the early sessions. In addition, she was counseled concerning sexual, needle sharing, and other behaviors that could transmit the virus to others or result in viral reexposure to herself. Other discussions emphasized the possible importance of maintaining good general health, eating nutritiously, and avoiding excessive use of alcohol or other chemical substances. The client was told that while definitive findings had not yet linked the maintenance of such general health behaviors to reduced likelihood of developing later illnesses by asymptomatic HIV-infected persons, it would be unwise to engage in activities that might compromise her immune system functioning.

In order to target her anxiety symptoms and provide a means to control anxiety without consuming intoxicants, the client was trained in progressive deep muscle relaxation using the standard Jacobsonian technique of tensing and relaxing 16 muscle groups. Two sessions of relaxation training were conducted during successive therapy visits, and the client was given a 30-minute audiotape recording of the relaxation instructions for daily home practice. Because sleep-onset insomnia and nightmares were among the symptoms she experienced, the client was instructed to practice the relaxation exercise in the evening before bedtime.

After 2 weeks of daily practice with progressive relaxation, the therapist trained the client in an abbreviated relaxation procedure and added cue-controlled relaxation. Rather than successively tense and relax each muscle group, the client was guided to direct her attention to each muscle group (hands, arms, shoulders, neck, forehead, face, jaw, upper and lower back, stomach, buttocks, thighs, calves, and feet) and "let go" of the tension present in the muscles as she breathed calmly and repeated, in thought, the word *calm* each time she exhaled. After relaxation had been induced in this manner, the therapist introduced a relaxing image that the client had previously identified (lying on the grass in a sunny meadow on a spring day) and instructed the client to"place" herself in thought within the relaxing imaginary scene. This exercise, which lasted about 20 minutes, was also audiotaped, and the client was provided with the tape for daily home practice over a 2-week period.

The client reported feelings of greater subjective relaxation during and immediately following each relaxation practice in the therapy sessions and at home. In order to extend the effects of relaxation, she was then encouraged to practice with the tape once each day and to set aside one or two 10-minute periods daily to practice the same exercise in a quiet location, but without the taped instructions. At first, the client was instructed to duplicate the full "letting go/cue-controlled/relaxing image" exercise just as it had been presented on the tape. She was then told that tension could be reduced in an even more abbreviated manner by closing her eyes, breathing calmly, covertly repeating the word *calm*, and relaxing any areas of her body that felt tense. The therapist suggested that the client use this technique any time she felt anxiety and to use the skill when she felt initial discomfort rather than waiting until anxiety became full-blown.

Relaxation training produced significant improvement in the client's reports of anxiety. However, because her anxiety was also mediated by cognitive and attributional factors, therapy sessions included attention to the client's cognitions and self-statement patterns, as discussed in the next section.

6.2.3. Interventions to Improve Cognitive Coping Skills

Careful assessment of cognitions, attitudes, labels, and attributions often reveals the presence of dysfunctional beliefs that elevate the HIV-exposed client's anxiety, depression, and distress. Broadly defined, these cognitive factors include the client's thoughts, self-statements, and evaluations about seropositivity; beliefs, interpretations, and attributions about HIV exposure and health; and cognitive reactions regarding how HIV exposure impacts on life. It would be highly unrealistic to expect persons not to worry if they learn that they are asymptomatic but HIV-infected, and, as discussed earlier, anxiety can motivate positive behavior change and evaluation of life values and goals. On the other hand, unalleviated rumination, obsessional or catastrophic thinking, and mis-construal of one's present health status can create great distress and interfere with adjustment. Among the most common dysfunctional cog-nitive patterns are misconceptions about the meaning of seropositivity (e.g., "This means I have AIDS"), health outlook ("I am going to die soon"), view of self ("I am infected and contaminated"), self-condemna-tion ("Why am I gay?" "I should never have used drugs. Why am I so stupid?"), and similar themes. Thoughts such as these are predictable after notification of seropositivity. However, if the client becomes debili-tated by them or experiences ongoing depression and anxiety that inter-fere with functioning, therapy to improve cognitive coping is warranted.

Several techniques can be implemented to help clients change maladaptive thought patterns that are recalcitrant to change through therapy discussion alone. The choice is probably best determined by each clinician's familiarity and skill with a particular technique. Established cognitive interventions that can be employed with HIV-seropositive persons include thought stopping (Wolpe, 1982), covert control and conditioning (Cautela & Bennett, 1981; Upper & Cautela, 1977), rational emotive therapy (Ellis, 1984; Ellis & Grieger, 1977; Ellis & Whitely, 1979), and cognitive therapy (Beck, 1976, Beck, Rush, Shaw, & Emery, 1979; Meichenbaum, 1977; Meichenbaum & Cameron, 1974). Although these approaches differ somewhat from one another, all are predicated on the assumption that thoughts influence feelings. By altering dysfunctional thoughts that trigger anxiety or depression, the client will be able to cope more effectively.

The purpose of thought stopping (Cautela & Wisocki, 1975; Wolpe, 1982) is to interrupt cognitions that precipitate maladaptive anxiety. It is often used in combination with anxiety-reduction methods. After identi-fying dysfunctional thoughts like those noted above, the therapist and the client together discuss the rationale for eliminating or controlling them. This discussion usually focuses around the fact that the identified self-statements have no value to the person and are actually detrimental because they lead to anxiety, depression, anger, social withdrawal, or self-deprecation. The therapist emphasizes the self-control aspect of the procedure, stressing that once the person has learned to use thought stopping, it remains available for use in the future.

Thought stopping in the treatment of an asymptomatic HIV-sero-positive client who catastrophizes that he has AIDS can be illustrated by the following therapy dialogue:

"Now sit back and relax, closing your eyes. In a few seconds, I'm going to say the word *begin*. I want you to deliberately think, *I've got AIDS*. As you begin the thought, signal me by raising your right index finger. Okay, lean back and relax. Are you ready? Begin."

As soon as the person raises a finger, the therapist loudly shouts, "*Stop*," producing a startled reaction. (In the case of highly anxious clients or those with cardiac problems, a less startling cue to stop should be used.) The client then opens his eyes and the therapist asks about the experience. Most clients respond, "You startled me," or "That scared me," or "You interrupted the thought." If the person does not mention spontaneously that the thought disappeared, then the therapist prompts that recognition and explains that a person cannot think of two things at the same time. Another trial is given and the therapist does not shout "Stop" immediately when the finger is raised but waits a second before evoking the startle response again. Again, after being asked about the experience, the person usually responds that the thought disappeared.

The client is then assisted in learning the technique as a self-management strategy without the therapist's direct intervention:

"Now, close your eyes again but this time I'm not going to shout, '*Stop*.' Try to imagine you hear yourself shouting *Stop* very loudly. Practice until you can imagine yourself as clearly and loudly as possible. Then open your eyes."

When the client does so, the therapist checks on the vividness of the imagery. If it was not sufficiently loud and clear to evoke a startle, the person is asked to practice again. If there continues to be a problem, the person is encouraged to yell, "Stop," several times during the therapy session and then to practice the technique again with the target thought (in this example, "I have AIDS"). The therapist and the client together practice interrupting the thought 15 to 20 times during the session until the person feels confident using the procedure. Between sessions, the client is instructed to practice thought stopping at planned intervals during the day and whenever the target thought recurs. During subsequent therapy sessions, 5 or 10 minutes may be devoted to additional thought-stopping practice.

Covert conditioning procedures (Upper & Cautela, 1977) are often combined with thought stopping and incorporate imagery into the intervention. After stopping a maladaptive thought, the client is instructed to take a deep breath and substitute for the maladaptive thought an incompatible and pleasant image. Using the example of a seropositive patient's recurrent troublesome thought "I've got AIDS," the procedure might be implemented by teaching the client to subvocally yell, "Stop," as described above, and then to slowly inhale and exhale while imagining a pleasant alternative. A client who is a recreational runner, for example, might be taught to visualize running along a quiet country road on a pleasant sunny day. The beautiful scenery is described in detail and a "runner's high" incorporated into the imagery, with the person feeling as though he could run forever, feeling healthy and vitally alive.

Thought stopping and covert conditioning are discrete, specific procedures that can be incorporated within the larger course of therapy with a client. There are also several broader cognitive therapy approaches that appear especially useful for clients whose depression, anxiety, and distress are worsened by recurrent maladaptive thoughts, beliefs, and attributions concerning HIV seropositivity. These approaches include the cognitive therapies of Beck (Beck, 1976; Beck *et al.*, 1979) and Meichenbaum (Meichenbaum, 1977; Meichenbaum & Cameron, 1974; Meichenbaum & Jaremko, 1983), and the rational emotive therapy (RET) model of Ellis (Ellis, 1984; Ellis & Grieger, 1977; Ellis & Whiteley, 1979). Both cognitive and RET approaches attempt to modify the client's anxiety-producing thoughts; they differ in the extent to which the therapist directly confronts the client's thoughts and attributional patterns, with RET more confrontive than cognitive therapy.

Beck, Meichenbaum, and other cognitive theorists assert that variables such as thoughts, labeling patterns, self-statements, and images are intimately related to dysfunctional behavior, and that distorted thought patterns can cause or maintain emotional maladjustment. Client cognitive distortions reflect unrealistic views of the world, future, and oneself that may seem illogical to others but are consistent with the client's own viewpoint. Cognitive distortions may be triggered by stressful life circumstances and are maintained by the client's style for judging and evaluating experiences.

Cognitive therapy begins with an assessment of the client's thoughts before or during periods of emotional upset. Because individuals are often unaware of their thoughts or "automatic" self-talk patterns, clients are often asked to self-monitor episodes of mood upset and to record the thought patterns that precede or accompany them. In the case of an anxious, asymptomatic, but HIV-seropositive client, the therapist should be particularly attuned to the presence of catastrophic thoughts ("I'm

worthless. No one will ever love me now"), exaggerated somatic preoccupation, and similar themes.

The goal of cognitive therapy is to assist clients in identifying when
they engage in maladaptive thoughts, interrupting those thoughts, and
substituting in their place self-statements which are more realistic and
which promote better coping. A variety of techniques are used to facilitate this process. One of the more common is for the therapist and the
client to generate a written list of statements that can serve as calming
alternatives to the present exaggerated, worrisome thoughts. For the
HIV-seropositive client preoccupied and incapacitated by the thought of
imminent death, these alternatives might emphasize that having HIV
antibodies is not the same as having AIDS, that the client will do everything possible to keep in good health, that worry is natural under the
circumstances but need not stop the client from living fully, and so on. In
therapy sessions and at home between sessions, clients are first asked to
read aloud these coping statements, then to practice repeating them in
thought, and, finally, to repeat them during times of impending emotional upset or in place of less adaptive thoughts. Detailed discussions of
the use of cognitive therapy techniques have been presented by several
theorists in this area (cf. Beck, 1976; Beck *et al.*, 1979; Meichenbaum,
1977).

The rational emotive therapy approach first outlined by Ellis (1984)
postulates that dysfunctional emotional consequences (C) result from an
interaction between some activating event (A) and the individual's
system of personal beliefs (B). While an activating event (such as
learning of HIV seropositivity) cannot be changed once it occurs, the
emotional consequence of that event to the individual is mediated by
beliefs, attributions, or other cognitive labeling processes that can be
influenced, controlled, and changed. Therapists using this approach can
help clients manage maladaptive symptoms by teaching them to
logically and rationally dispute (D) incorrect, unreasonable, or
unrealistic beliefs. Following an educational period in which the
therapist teaches the client about the model (often presented in an A-B-
C-D schematic fashion), the therapist prompts the client to retain
reasonable thoughts but change those irrational beliefs that currently
contribute to distress. Using the example discussed earlier, an
asymptomatic but HIV-infected client incapacitated by fear of death
might be taught to logically challenge the fear-producing belief ("I will

get AIDS and die") with other beliefs, such as "I am in good health now," "HIV positive is not the same as AIDS," "I wish I didn't have the virus, but I am going to use the knowledge to do everything possible to live healthfully," or "I will keep myself in the best shape I can because there are certain to be medical advances in this area over the next few years." As in the cognitive therapy approaches, therapists using RET often ask clients to self-monitor negative affective states and their accompanying cognitive patterns. Clients may also be given "cue cards" or other prompting devices with written "rational thoughts" to read when troublesome thoughts or mood upsets occur between sessions.

The detrimental effect of dysfunctional cognitions on adjustment and future health are well documented (Affleck, Tennen, Croog, & Levine, 1987; Cousins, 1979; Janoff-Bulman & Frieze, 1983; Silver & Wortman, 1980; Taylor, 1980). Causal attributions affect future health by influencing perceptions of control and predictability, which in turn motivate adaptive behavior change (Affleck *et al.*, 1987; Krantz & Deckel, 1983). Cardiac patients' causal attributions, for example, influence whether they subsequently adopt health-promoting regimens; persons who attribute illness to random chance are less likely to adhere to behavior-change programs than those who perceive control over their circumstances (Affleck *et al.*, 1987; Cousins, 1979; Janoff-Bulman & Frieze, 1983; Silver & Wortman, 1980; Taylor, 1980). The perception of control is also related to whether or not patients follow medical advice following the diagnosis of physical illness (Brownlee-Duffeck *et al.*, 1987; Mitchell & Stuart, 1984; Plotkin-Israel, 1984). Thus, cognitive factors can influence both future health course and the manner in which a person adjusts to a health-threatening experience (Brownlee-Duffeck *et al.*, 1987; Hammen, Jacobs, Mayol, & Cochran, 1980; Hazaleus & Deffenbacher, 1986).

The therapeutic use of cognitive coping strategies with an HIV-positive client is illustrated in the following case example.

6.2.3.1. Case Example

A 32-year-old HIV-seropositive homosexual male was referred for therapy by his physician after he developed symptoms of anxiety, depression, and somatization. The client learned that he was HIV-seropositive approximately 1 year earlier and had a number of friends who had died of AIDS-related illnesses. After learning of his seropositivity, the client consulted his physician frequently with complaints of tension headaches, leg pains, and nonspecific feelings of illness. However, repeated medical evaluations revealed no clinical evidence of any HIV illness, and all laboratory tests of T-cell counts, cerebrospinal fluid, and skin-test allergic reactivity were normal. Psychological factors were believed to be responsible for his symptoms.

During initial visits, the client reported preoccupation with his sero-positivity, frequent ruminations that he would become ill and die within days or weeks, sleep disturbance, and social withdrawal. He focused vigilant attention on any body discomfort and attributed even transient discomforts to the onset of AIDS. The client reported depressed mood, frequent crying episodes, and occasional suicidal thoughts. Although he did not have a steady relationship partner, the client had supportive friends and maintained his professional employment. However, he be-came increasingly avoidant of others and reported that frequent anger and irritability at work were jeopardizing his employment. When asked by the therapist how he felt about himself, the client said he was "con-taminated" and viewed his body fluids as "poison."

Because it appeared that much of the individual's psychological dis-tress, social avoidance, and somatization were a result of his cognitions and attributions, intervention first focused on this area. The therapist discussed with the client how thoughts and self-statements influence emotions, adjustment, and self-appraisal, and the client was encouraged to view self-statements as determinants of his own mood. For a 2-week period, the client was asked to monitor his emotional state, recording on a 0-to-100 intensity scale his depression or upset during any particularly emotional periods. He recorded thoughts associated with each episode by writing, in as detailed a manner as possible, what he was thinking immediately before the episode as well as what he did immediately after the distressing episode. These monitoring records, reviewed by the therapist, revealed that virtually all depressive periods were preceded by a variety of cognitions emphasizing fatalism ("I'm going to die"), help-lessness ("There's nothing I can do to get rid of the virus in my system"), perceived similarity by himself to AIDS patients he had known ("John learned he was HIV-positive, developed AIDS, and then had a horrible death"), and somatic preoccupations ("I don't think I feel well. I wonder if this is the start of pneumonia or something"). Most depressed episodes lasted for hours, were accompanied by many such ruminations, and usu-ally ended only when he eventually fell asleep or became intoxicated.

During an early session, the therapist provided the client with accu-rate information concerning HIV seropositivity, emphasizing distinctions between his asymptomatic status and AIDS. While "pat" reassurances in such situations are inappropriate and unwarranted, the client was told that the probability was high that he would remain in good health for years. Because the client had been sexually abstinent for over 1 year and was already highly knowledgeable about risk precautions, substantial counseling concerning sexuality was not necessary.

Following the procedures of Meichenbaum (1977) and Beck (1976), the therapist and the client developed written lists of self-statements that could be used to replace the maladaptive cognitions that were instigating and exacerbating his anxiety and depression. Some alternative statements involved disputations of the client's worrisome, but incorrect, ruminations ("I have been exposed to the virus, but I don't have AIDS" and "I am in good health; there's nothing wrong with my body"). Other alternative self-statements emphasized reattributions concerning minor aches and pains ("I guess I'm tired today, but it's because I didn't get to bed early. I'll feel better when I get to work") and themes involving self-efficacy ("I'll keep myself in the best health possible." "I wish this hadn't happened, but I am not going to let it control my life"). Initially, the client practiced reading aloud the list of alternative statements at home and in therapy sessions, attending closely to the meaning of each statement as he read it. During times of incipient rumination, he was taught to thought-stop and then to speak aloud or say covertly the same kinds of statements. Although the actual generation of alternative statements and the overt or covert practice in repeating them required little time, therapy to help the client change self-talk and attributional patterns required several months. In addition to cognitive modification therapy, the therapist worked with the client to make other behavior changes, such as spending less time alone at night when ruminations usually occurred, planning weekly goals for socializing and becoming involved in recreational activities, and reducing tension in ways other than intoxicant overuse.

6.2.4. Interventions to Improve Social Functioning

As described in the previous chapter, it is common for persons to react to seropositivity by social withdrawal and self-isolation. In part, this may be secondary to depression, anxiety, anger, and other psychological difficulties that interfere with interest in social and other activities. The problem can be confounded when persons who previously provided dependable support distance themselves from the HIV-affected individual. In extreme cases, the authors have known HIV-seropositive persons who have left their jobs and isolated themselves at home, waiting to die from AIDS. While these latter reactions are extreme, the social isolation and withdrawal that follow HIV seropositivity are quite common.

It can be particularly therapeutic to help the HIV-positive person to reinstate gratifying activities that were enjoyed in the past but were discontinued after the person learned of HIV exposure. Intervention focuses upon living fully and responsibly rather than overemphasizing the possibility of future disease progression. Another useful therapeutic strategy is to explore the client's hopes for the future and to orient the client toward planning for life rather than preparing for death. Learning that they are HIV-infected, even if in good present health, almost inevitably leads clients to become aware of their own mortality. HIV seropositivity can provide the impetus to proceed with plans, goals, and aspirations now rather than deferring them until some indeterminant future date. Obviously, judgment must be exercised to ensure that the specific goals are reasonable and likely to enhance life satisfaction, rather than generate other problems. However, knowledge of HIV seropositivity can be the stimulus for constructive life changes. The authors have known persons who made constructive job changes, developed business and creative interests based upon previously undeveloped talent, became involved in community service and political activities, and learned skills that were a source of pride and pleasure after seropositivity. In the process, problems with social isolation often abate.

Many HIV-seropositive persons, especially those who are gay or are involved in drug use subcultures, have alternative life-styles that are outside the traditional mainstream of American society. The upset resulting from HIV seropositivity can produce further isolation, not only from the larger society but also from the networks that had formerly provided support. These include general friend, social support, and social activity networks, as well as relationships with family members and significant others.

6.2.4.1. Engagement in Social Supports

As discussed in Chapter 5, disclosure of seropositivity to others can serve to mobilize support and can assist the psychologically distressed client to cope more successfully (Zones *et al.*, 1987). On the other hand, disclosure can also carry highly negative ramifications that complicate client adjustment owing to social stigma, fear, and discrimination potential. Therapists should take into account the nature of a client's relationships, the probable response of others to knowledge that the client is seropositive, the familiarity of others with HIV infection and AIDS, ethical obligations, and prevailing attitudes toward AIDS when discussing the potential benefits and risks if the client were to disclose his or her HIV status to friends, family members, and others.

Clients who have responded to knowledge of seropositivity in a self-withdrawing and insular manner can benefit from attention to improving social supports. Larger cities often have support groups specifically for persons coping with seropositivity; these programs may be offered by AIDS service organizations, progressive church organizations, and community clinics. Responsibly conducted support groups are of great potential value because they allow the client to share feelings and concerns with understanding others, to feel less "alone," and to learn styles of coping along with people who face the same adjustment issues. As the magnitude of the health crisis expands, there will be an increased need for support groups of this kind.

It may, under some circumstances, be necessary to counsel HIV-seropositive clients toward different support networks than they had in the past. Sadly, and especially in areas outside the nation's largest cities, persons whose HIV status becomes known may still find themselves shunned by friends, acquaintances, co-workers, and others. In other cases, it is in the client's interest to develop new activities and support networks. An HIV-seropositive former intravenous drug user whose friends are drug users, the problem-drinker client, or the individual used to a "fast lane" sexual life-style may benefit from assistance in the development of new social supports, activities, and pursuits.

6.2.4.2. Relationships with Family and Significant Others

As we discussed in the previous chapter, persons differ markedly in their reaction to knowledge that a member of their family is HIV-infected. Under the most ideal of circumstances, family members will respond in supportive, understanding ways. Often, however, parents, children, brothers, sisters, and other relatives share the same fears and misconceptions about AIDS as the general public and may be very uncomfortable with the seropositive client. While some family members are directly rejecting of the seropositive individuals, we more frequently observe ambivalence: attempts to be supportive but with fears about casual contagion; discomfort with client life-style, especially if the client is homosexual or bisexual; avoidance of the client but guilt concerning it;

and concern for the client but also concern that the family will be stigmatized if others learn that a member is affected by the virus that causes AIDS.

Therapy with family members of the client may enable them to cope more effectively with their own feelings and relate more effectively with the client. One aspect of consultation with family members is information provision, including an explanation of the meaning of antibody-positive status, differentiation of asymptomatic infection from AIDS, alleviating concerns about virus transmission during everyday household contact, and related information. However, family members may also require more comprehensive therapy assistance as they attempt to deal with their fears, anger, guilt, and feelings toward the client.

Finally, the emotional needs of the spouse or relationship partner of an HIV client are often substantial and, too often, are neglected. Spouses of hemophiliacs or transfusion recipients, heterosexual relationship partners, spouses of intravenous drug users, women married to husbands who acquired HIV infection through bisexual behavior, and homosexual lovers of gay men with HIV infection are some of the traditional and nontraditional spouses and spouse-equivalents who are directly affected by a client's HIV seropositivity. Invariably, relationship partners must confront not only their fears for the other person but also fear concerning their own health. Depending upon the couple's skills for coping with stress, other relationship problems may develop and merit couple therapy intervention. While the event precipitating couple stress—one member's HIV seropositivity—may be different from the usual basis for couple difficulties, and while the couple relationship may be nontraditional, it is likely that standard marital therapy and communication/problem-solving approaches (cf. Gottman, Notarious, Gonso, & Hartman, 1979; Jacobson & Margolin, 1979; Stuart, 1980) can be adapted for intervention in this area.

6.2.4.3. Case Example

This 45-year-old homosexual male learned of his HIV seropositivity after he voluntarily sought antibody testing from his physician. In much the same way as the other case examples described in this chapter, the client experienced a period of shock and disbelief immediately after learning of his antibody status. Gradually, he developed symptoms of anxiety, depression, and somatization. In addition, he gradually withdrew from others. The client reported that when he confided his HIV-antibody status to some friends, they became distant and uncomfortable and avoided further contact with him. Although he expected this response from some of his heterosexual acquaintances, some of the gay men in his social network were equally nonsupportive and avoidant. Gradually, the client removed himself from social outlets and declined invitations even from others who still included him in their social activities. When he sought therapy, the client had withdrawn from most of his social supports. He continued to work but stayed alone in his home each night and was preoccupied with feelings of impending death even though he was without any symptoms of illness. It was the therapist's impression that the client had withdrawn from others, held fears that he might "contaminate" them, and became more absorbed in planning for his death than in living in the present.

If there had been a social support group for HIV-seropositive persons in his city, involvement in it would have been a logical part of the intervention. Unfortunately, there was no such group, and the therapist felt it would be unwise for this client to become involved in activities for persons with AIDS or advanced HIV-related illnesses since that might worsen rather than alleviate his distress. Consequently, the therapist saw the client individually, but with the aims of alleviating his depression and countering his social withdrawal.

Initial sessions focused on changing many of the same cognitive and rumination patterns discussed in the preceding case study. After rapport with the client had been established, the therapist also began to directly confront some aspects of the client's self-defeating behavior. In particular, the client was encouraged to view his withdrawal, preoccupation with death, and self-imposed isolation as patterns that interfered with living. The therapist behaviorally contracted with the client to spend time outside of his home and in the company of others. At first, the goals were modest: Going to a movie with a friend or inviting someone for dinner were the initial weekly activities. The client was encouraged to socialize with persons who had been supportive and had attempted to initiate contact even after they learned of his HIV status rather than those who seemed to avoid him. As therapy continued, attention focused on other ways to establish a broader social support network in which the client would feel comfortable and accepted. The therapist discussed community groups where he might feel comfortable even if his HIV status were known, including an existing gay community AIDS education program and the local Metropolitan Community Church, which served a predominantly homosexual congregation. The client agreed to attend one meeting of each organization during the week after the therapy session took place. In the following session, he reported feeling particularly welcomed at the church, where he met several people and was invited to a church-sponsored supper.

The client also reported that he had particularly enjoyed dancing in the past, although he had not done so for some time. The client was assisted in planning for small group outings to a local dance club. During later visits, it became apparent to the therapist that the client was establishing friendships and was increasingly involved in his new supportive network. When therapy terminated after about eight visits, the client said that he was planning to continue these activities but planned to remain sexually abstinent in order to prevent any possibility that he would transmit HIV infection to others or become reexposed himself.

6.3. OTHER CONSIDERATIONS

Individuals who are HIV-seropositive, even if in good health, face inevitable anxieties and fears about the future. Therapy, no matter how skillful and sensitive, cannot remove fundamental uncertainties about future health raised when a person learns that he or she has been infected with the human immunodeficiency virus. A proportion of HIV-infected persons will develop serious illnesses within 5 years of the time of their exposure. However, a greater proportion will not, at least over this time period. While therapy interventions cannot provide answers to unanswerable questions about a client's long-term health, clients can be helped to cope constructively with anxiety and to live fully in spite of it. The longer that HIV-seropositive persons remain in good health, the greater will be their opportunity to benefit from forthcoming medical advances in the management, treatment, and prevention of the more serious HIV diseases.

All of the intervention approaches discussed in this chapter were developed prior to the AIDS health crisis and none were originally intended for counseling persons distressed upon learning of their HIV seropositivity. However, because these therapy methods have proven effective for treating similar adjustment problems, they also merit the attention of therapists who see clients coping with their HIV status. As therapists and researchers direct greater attention to the mental health needs of HIV-seropositive persons, more individual and group counseling intervention approaches will be identified and evaluated.

Psychological Consequences of AIDS and AIDS-Related Complex

The strongest predictor of developing an HIV-related disease is the amount of time that has elapsed since viral exposure (Moss *et al.*, 1987). Even if HIV transmission rates could be stopped immediately or a vaccine were quickly developed, the number of new ARC and AIDS cases will continue to increase for years to come since millions of persons are already infected with the virus. From 10 to 43% of HIV-seropositive persons develop AIDS within 5 years after infection, with increasing risk over time (Collier, Murphy, Roberts, & Handsfield, 1987; Lange *et al.*, 1987; Moss *et al.*, 1987). In light of these estimates, an additional 700,000 persons can be predicted to require treatment for ARC and AIDS within the next 5 years.

In this chapter, we will examine the factors that influence a person's adjustment to an ARC or AIDS diagnosis and then discuss common psychological consequences that follow these diagnoses. While the consequences to the individual affected by ARC or AIDS are devastating, the diagnoses create distress as well to lovers, family members, friends, and health care providers. This chapter will also consider the impact of these illnesses upon significant others and caregivers, in addition to the patient.

As discussed in Chapter 1, AIDS-related complex (ARC) is an "umbrella" label for a host of different physical illnesses. The ARC patient may experience mild and transient symptoms of immunocompromise, or may become extremely ill and die even though the illness does not meet the definitional requirements of clinical criterion AIDS. It is estimated that at least 17 to 25% of the individuals infected with HIV will eventually develop ARC symptoms (Levine et al., 1987). Some investigators describe ARC as a mild form of AIDS (Ziegler & Abrams, 1985), while others regard it as a prodromal stage before the later development of AIDS (Mathur-Wagh et al., 1984). Although patients may only have symptoms of persistent generalized lymphadenopathy or even become asymptomatic and seemingly well, persistent ARC symptoms are an unfavorable prognostic sign for the later development of AIDS (Visscher et al., 1987). The specific determinants of disease progression are not yet known. As mentioned earlier, a number of possible cofactors for illness development have been implicated. These include the use of other immunosuppressant substances (Goedert, 1985; Jaffe et al., 1983; Marmor et al., 1982), reexposure to multiple strains of the virus (Ciobanu & Wiernik, 1986; Drew, 1986; Sonnabend et al., 1985), or even possible genetic determinants that mediate HIV susceptibility (Eales et al., 1987).

ARC often carries a frustrating and unpredictable health course. Patients may feel quite well and healthy one day but become quite ill the next. Although most physicians are now well educated about the signs of full-blown AIDS, the symptoms of ARC are more subtle and diffuse. Because these early symptoms are less identifiable, they may be discounted by both the physician and the patient when they first appear. More than half of persons with ARC dismiss their early symptoms as being of little consequence and do not seek out medical care (Mandel, 1985; Mandel & Namir, 1986; Mandel, Coates, Wiley, Bart, & Woods, 1987), often waiting more than 8 months before seeing a physician. Because the many illnesses that constitute ARC are diverse and often subtle, specific diagnostic conclusions may be difficult to reach.

There are many uncertainties associated with ARC, and while some illnesses are quite treatable, it is not possible to predict a definitive, long-term response to medical treatment. ARC patients often do not qualify for disability payments or unemployment compensation, even though Mandel, Coates, et al., (1987) found that half of the ARC patients in their sample were sufficiently handicapped to cause unemployability. Thus, the person with ARC may be too sick to work but, in the absence of an AIDS diagnosis, are ineligible for assistance to replace lost wages.

Full-blown or frank AIDS has devastating psychological consequences since it is almost invariably fatal. While 80% of persons diagnosed with AIDS die within 2 years of diagnosis (Curran *et al.*, 1985), these mortality data disguise the variable clinical course of persons with AIDS. Some individuals experience sudden disease onset and die within a short time from a particularly virulent illness. Others may be extremely ill, but recover from an initial episode and remain relatively healthy until the next acute illness. A small percentage of AIDS patients enter periods of remission and remain seemingly healthy for periods of time that exceed the statistical averages. There is no single health course that applies uniformly to all persons with AIDS.

7.1. FACTORS INFLUENCING PSYCHOLOGICAL REACTIONS TO AN ARC OR AIDS DIAGNOSIS

Many factors have been identified that mediate psychological reactions to an ARC or AIDS diagnosis. These include persons' health status and symptom severity, attributions regarding their illness, self-disclosure of health problems, familiarity with the disease, and available environmental supports.

7.1.1. Health Status

As would be expected, the severity of the illness influences a person's reaction to an ARC or AIDS diagnosis. Persons with ARC have a particularly difficult time with anxiety as they cope with the possibility of future health problems. For AIDS patients, their youth and the lethality of the diagnosis precipitate a sudden confrontation with all of the complex existential and personal issues of death and dying . Persons who are extremely ill may surrender any effort to recover, passively waiting for death. Other are tenacious in their efforts to recover and "live with AIDS," rather than die from AIDS.

7.1.2. Attributions Regarding Illness

A patient's attributions or beliefs regarding the cause of the illness can influence the extent to which the person will experience emotional distress. Patients typically attempt to find some meaning for their altered health and search for explanations in their past choices and actions. In a study of gay and bisexual men with AIDS (Moulton, Sweet, Temoshok, & Mandel, 1987) found that 78% of AIDS patients attributed their illnesses to their own behavior. Such self-attributions engendered greater distress than external attributions, such as believing the illness to be accidental or simple bad luck. Among ARC patients, the pattern was reversed, with self-attribution associated with less distress. Persons who believed they were responsible for their illnesses also believed they could influence their future health. ARC patients who believed they could make healthy life-style changes such as improved diet, stress reduction, and exercise experienced considerably less distress. Thus, for ARC patients, self-attributions were associated with a belief in a self-efficacy. This suggests that the belief that one can influence the course of the illness, with its attendant perception of personal control, may differentiate ARC patients who develop severe psychosocial reactions from those who react constructively to their illness.

As yet, there has been no research that compares the attributions made by different AIDS patient populations regarding their illness. However, Brondolo, Clemow, Saidi, and Lerner (1987) conducted a psychosocial needs assessment with hemophiliac patients and their families. Since 90% of the hemophiliacs who received blood products between 1978 and 1985 are HIV-exposed, this group would be predicted to display high levels of distress. However, both the hemophiliac patients and their family members reported relatively low levels of distress. Brondolo et al., (1987) speculate that hemophilia patients may have developed effective coping skills from years of dealing with a serious illness. Another reason for the difference between the distress levels of gay patients in the Moulton et al., study (1987) and the hemophiliacs in the Brondolo et al. project (1987) may be a function of their different attributions. While the gay men attributed their illness to personal life-style choices and the decision to engage in sexual behavior that transmitted the virus, hemophiliacs were more likely to believe they were the "accidental" victims of an unforeseeable, and therefore unpreventable, chance occurrence in the course of their medical care. Thus, the gay men were more likely to evidence self-blame, while hemophiliacs were more likely to hold more external attributions.

7.1.3. Reactions to the Diagnosis

Mandel and Namir (1986) conducted a longitudinal psychosocial study at the University of California, San Francisco, in part to assess how patients react to being diagnosed with ARC or AIDS. When patients diagnosed with either AIDS, acute leukemia, or malignant melanoma were compared, similar reaction patterns were evidenced by the three patient groups over a 2-month postdiagnostic period. All three groups demonstrated clinically significant increases in anxiety and depression and were not significantly different from one another on measures of self-esteem or locus of control. The most prevalent postdiagnostic concerns expressed by patients in all three groups were fears regarding prolonged illness, fears of becoming dependent or burdening others, and fears of dying. There are typical human responses to life-threatening illnesses. The Mandel and Namir (1986) findings suggest that health providers can extrapolate from the wide body of existing literature on adjustments to other life-threatening illnesses to guide their clinical interventions with ARC and AIDS patients until more specific knowledge emerges.

7.1.4. Self-Disclosure of Health Problems

Upon learning of seropositivity, and again when physical symptoms appear, the HIV-affected person faces the dilemma of whether to discuss these health problems with others. Social supports play an important role in coping with other life-threatening illnesses, suggesting that self-disclosure can often secure emotional support from others and promote adaptive coping. In fact, receiving social support has been identified as the single most helpful resource by persons with all stages of HIV infection (Coates, Stall, et al., 1987).

Gay men who are comfortable with their identity are more likely to have previously disclosed their sexual preference to others (Cass, 1979). Several researchers suggest that prior disclosure about sexual identity may be associated with a more positive adjustment after an ARC or AIDS diagnosis for gay men (Morin, Charles, & Malyon, 1984). This makes intuitive sense because, in disclosing homosexual preferences, the person may have developed communication skills and coping strategies for disclosing personal information. Mandel, Coates, et al., (1987) reported that not having "come out" as a homosexual was the most frequently cited reason for also not disclosing AIDS-related health problems to others. However, many gay men who have formerly disclosed their sexual preference to others still do not share their health problems with friends or family, or in the workplace. While 80% of the men in Mandel's study had disclosed their homosexuality to family or co-workers before becoming diagnosed with ARC or AIDS, many had not discussed their health problems with either family or co-workers 2 months following diagnosis.

The same investigators (Mandel, 1985; Mandel, Coates, et al., 1987) also found that gay men who disclosed their health status to others reported less emotional distress than persons who had withheld this information from others. However, the effects of disclosing that one had ARC or AIDS clearly depend upon the social responses of the persons to whom this information is disclosed. Mandel found that when negative reactions from others followed disclosure, the already significant stress of coping with the disease was exacerbated. For some persons, disclosure of an AIDS-related illness may involve revealing other previously undisclosed information about stigmatized life-style, such as drug use or homosexuality (Coates, Stall, et al., 1987). Under these conditions, disclosure can exacerbate the person's distress rather than mobilize support. As a result, many persons, with ARC and AIDS elect not to disclose their health status to significant others, fearing that this information will lead to rejection instead of emotional support (Coates, Stall, et al., 1987; Mandel, Coates, et al., 1987; Mandel & Namir, 1986). Impediments to disclosure include fear of job loss, fear of physical attack or emotional estrangement, fear of stressing family relationships, fear of losing health insurance benefits, and dealing with others' fear of contagion.

These findings have several implications for clinicians. Individuals who have previously disclosed potentially stigmatizing information, such as drug use or homosexuality, may have greater skill or comfort in self-disclosing personally relevant and difficult information to others. Persons who have withheld information about their AIDS-related health problems or who received negative reactions following disclosure of their illnesses can be expected to exhibit greater distress than those whose health disclosures mobilize social or relationship supports. Gay men who have not previously disclosed their homosexuality and who now also confront the problems associated with ARC or AIDS may be at the highest risk for severe emotional distress. The simultaneous disclosure that one has AIDS and is gay or uses drugs can precipitate major difficulties and anxiety. In additions, patients who receive rejection and hostility will have their health adjustment complicated by negative reactions from those they had hoped would become a source of support.

7.1.5. Availability of Environmental Support Systems

Social support is clearly pivotal to persons attempting to cope with serious illnesses. Individuals with many potential supports and resources to draw upon are better able to replace those supports that are lost if some people distance themselves following the diagnosis. No existing research has compared the distress of persons in geographical areas with extensive support services with those of persons in areas where few resources exist. However, it is likely that persons who can turn to alternative supports and resources are in a better position to develop coping skills and replace lost support networks. The extent and availability of such services differ widely across the country. As a general rule, large cities most hard-hit by the health crisis have developed greater   social assistance and supports, while areas with low to moderate AIDS prevalence have fewer available organized resources.

7.2. PSYCHOLOGICAL CONSEQUENCES OF ARC AND AIDS

The psychosocial suffering of persons with ARC and AIDS occurs on several levels. On a physical level, individuals face adjustment to the illness. This may include extreme alterations in energy and physical health, pain, breathlessness, disfigurement, or changes in body image. On the psychological level, intense anxiety, depression, helplessness, hopelessness, isolation, anger, and cognitive deterioration are common. And, on a social level, the individual faces possible disruption in relationships, employment, discrimination, housing, income, and financial status. Taken together, these changes can be devastating for the person with AIDS, as well as to others in his or her social and family network. As the severity of symptoms and illness increase, psychological distress often increases correspondingly. Tross *et al.* (1987) found that 52% of persons with AIDS and 64% of persons with ARC displayed common and highly treatable adverse psychological reactions. While all patients do not experience extreme emotional distress (Mandel, 1985), such reactions are sufficiently common to suggest that mental health and social support services should be made available to all patients with AIDS and ARC.

7.2.1. Anxiety

Many studies find that ARC patients are even more distressed than persons with AIDS (Abrams, Dilley, Maxey, & Volberding, 1986; Temoshok, Sweet, Moulton, & Zich, 1987). Given the ambiguity and uncertainty engendered by an ARC diagnosis, persons with ARC experience high levels of anxiety regarding their future health and fears of developing AIDS. The appearance and lessening of ARC symptoms can precipitate relief as a symptom ameliorates, but intense anxiety as another symptom appears. This fluctuating cycle often repeats itself with each slight physical change.

Some ARC patients who develop AIDS experience transient relief following the AIDS diagnosis (Abrams *et al.*, 1986), probably because the diagnosis alleviates the uncertainty with which they have lived. However, such relief may be temporary. Psychological symptoms reappear and, understandably, 90% of persons with AIDS report experiencing fear and anxiety (Grady, Jacob, Baird, Spross, & Ostchega, 1987). In the later disease stages, anxiety shifts from anticipating disease progression to anticipating death and dying. Patients often fear the possibility of extreme life-sustaining measures, which compromise their dignity, and fear the possibility of a lingering, prolonged death or disfigurement before their death. It is common for patients to begin an existential contemplation of their lives, the significance of death, and the meaning of life itself.

Not all persons with AIDS were diagnosed with ARC before receiving the AIDS diagnosis. The AIDS patient who has not dealt with earlier stages of HIV-related disease may have the most difficult time adjusting to the illness since all of these issues occur simultaneously. Some patients want to discuss their feelings about the illness at length. Others will resist acknowledging them at all.

7.2.2. Depression

Depression and anxiety are the most common psychological reactions following a diagnosis of AIDS or ARC. Isolation may result when the diagnosed person withdraws from others or when existing social support networks withdraw from the person following his or her diagnosis. Many newly diagnosed persons anticipate negative reactions from others and act self-protectively so as to forestall these anticipated negative reactions for as long as possible. More than half of persons with ARC and AIDS express fear about others' reactions, and one-third maintain silence rather than risk personal rejection until the symptoms make it impossible to maintain any pretense of normality (Pollak, Gharakhanian, *et al.*, 1987). The obvious disadvantage of self-isolation and nondisclosure is that the person simultaneously lessens any possibility of receiving emotional support or understanding. While such self-imposed isolation protects the person from adverse reactions, it also excludes supportive responses and can, therefore, contribute to depression.

In some areas such as San Francisco, persons with ARC or AIDS anticipated adverse reactions from others that were exaggerated well beyond the reactions they actually received (Stempel *et al.*, 1987). Supportive responses occurred more often than they had been expected and became an important source of emotional support. However, these results may be a function of the area of the country in which the study was conducted and less likely to occur in small-town middle America. Reports of supportive reactions tend to emanate from areas of the country that have substantial experience with the AIDS epidemic and where many people have been personally affected by the health crisis. Affirmation and emotional support are more unlikely in areas of the country that have less experience with the disease and where misinformation is more rampant.

Social support helps individuals cope with major life crises, yet many AIDS-affected persons report reductions in social support from lovers, friends, and family (Bechtel, 1987). These patient self-reports are confirmed by a project in which researchers at New York's Montefiore Hospital studied the effects of an AIDS diagnosis on social interactions between AIDS patients and their family members. Friedland, Kahl, *et al.* (1987) evaluated the sharing of household facilities and close personal interactions between household contacts and persons with AIDS both before and after the AIDS diagnosis. Detailed standardized interviews were administered to family members to determine the nature and frequency of their household interactions with the person with AIDS. The results indicated that major and significant reductions in sharing and physical contact followed the diagnosis. Personal contact, such as hugs or kisses on the cheek, decreased markedly after diagnosis. The sharing of common household items, such as eating utensils, plates, or towels, decreased following the diagnosis, and family members evidenced reluctance to continue sharing bathrooms or bedrooms with the AIDS patient. Thus, there is support for individuals' fears that they may experience rejection from the significant people in their lives.

Pollak, Gharakhanian, *et al.* (1987) researched the self-isolation that often follows an AIDS diagnosis and found that not all AIDS patients maintained their silence out of fear. Some patients refused to seek psychological support from others and carried on with their lives just as they had before receiving the diagnosis. They maintained hope by maintaining their usual daily routines, reluctant to modify their lives or attend to their diagnosis. Pollak, Gharakhanian, *et al.* (1987) point out that this response creates a double bind. On the one hand, refusing to orient daily life around illness can preserve optimism for the future (Bickelhaupt, 1986). Abrams *et al.* (1986) suggest that such responses may be adaptive, and there is some empirical support for their contention. Research with patients facing other terminal illnesses found that "successful denial" is associated not only with lower anxiety and maintaining hope but also with greater longevity following diagnosis (Hackett & Cassem, 1970; Hackett & Weisman, 1969). But it also sets up a potential problem, since the person cannot receive emotional support during those times when it is needed if significant others are unaware of the person's uncommunicated emotional needs.

7.2.3. Anger

Persons with ARC and AIDS also experience anger over their diagnosis (Feinblum, 1986; Temoshok, Sweet, *et al.*, 1987; U.S. Department of Health and Human Services, 1986b). Grady *et al.* (1987) report that 83% of AIDS patients admit to difficulty managing their anger. While anger is a common experience, the reasons for it differ from person to person. Some react to feeling victimized by a virus or experience anger toward those who may have transmitted the virus to them. Uncaring reactions and social insensitivity may be encountered and contribute to the problem (Joseph, 1986). One person with AIDS described his increasing frustration and anger by noting, "I looked for options and found only barriers." The inability of healthcare providers to provide solutions and cures becomes another source of frustration (Eisdorfer, 1987b). And many patients experience periods when they are angry with themselves for engaging in behavior that exposed them to viral infection. Cohen and Weisman (1986) followed 300 persons with AIDS and ARC over time and reported a consistent theme of alienation, frustration, and anger.

7.3. NEUROPSYCHOLOGICAL CONSEQUENCES OF ARC AND AIDS

At first, organic brain syndromes observed in some AIDS patients were thought to be secondary to other opportunistic infections. The evidence is now clear that HIV is neurotropic as well as lymphotropic and directly invades the central nervous system to produce changes in neurological functioning (Epstein, Shorer, Cho, Murphy-Corb, & Baskin, 1987; Eskin & Stoler, 1987; Ruff et al., 1987). In a study by Leiderman et al. (1985), HIV was isolated from the cerebrospinal fluid of all AIDS patients with encephalopathies. It is estimated that 30 to 75% of persons with AIDS eventually develop neurological complications (Levy et al., 1985; Snider et al., 1983; Wolcott, 1986b) and that 70% of AIDS patients show evidence of CNS disease by the time of death (Levy et al., 1985). Navia and Price (1986) report that 67% of AIDS patients revealed autopsy evidence of a premortem AIDS dementia and that 25% had neurological symptoms even before their AIDS diagnosis. Other researchers have confirmed that CNS involvement frequently antedates the development of AIDS (Siegal et al., 1987).

The variety of acute and chronic organic mental states and central nervous system (CNS) diseases found among persons with ARC and AIDS is diverse, and neurological invasion can be reflected by myriad symptoms. Depending upon the specific disease and process, persons with AIDS may display neurological and behavioral signs and symptoms that are diffuse or focal, acute or chronic (Coates, Stall, et al., 1987; Levy et al., 1985; Siegal et al., 1987; Snider et al., 1983; Wolcott, 1986b).

The most widely described neurological syndrome has been called "AIDS dementia," "subacute encephalitis," or "AIDS encephalopathy" (Coates, Stall, et al., 1987). While the syndrome has not yet been fully characterized, it shares many features in common with the subcortical dementias (Sidtis, Amitai, Ornitz, & Price, 1987). Primary AIDS dementia has a gradual and progressive onset (Eisdorfer, 1987b). Since the initial symptoms mimic psychological reactions, differential diagnosis is difficult, especially in the early stages of neurological involvement. Neuropsychological examination of patients across the spectrum of HIV infection ranging from asymptomatic HIV infection to ARC to frank AIDS indicates significant and progressive decrements in performance across these patient groups. As severity of HIV infection increases, neurological impairments become increasingly evident (Sidtis et al., 1987). Early symptoms may include memory and concentration difficulties, motor slowing, bilateral leg weakness, problems with coordination and balance, and an unsteady gait (Eisdorfer, 1987b; Sidtis et al., 1987). Early behavioral signs of dementia include social withdrawal, apathy, irritability, decreased spontaneity, and an overall slowing in daily functioning (Holland & Tross, 1985; Navia & Price, 1986; Sidtis *et al.*, 1987). Since these symptoms are also common in depression, it can be difficult to differentiate functional depressive reactions from the early signs of dementia (Holland & Tross, 1985; Navia & Price, 1986; Wolcott, 1986b).

Over time, and if dementia progresses, more global cognitive impairments can occur. The patient may evidence more impulsivity, impaired judgment, and increased difficulty in organizing and carrying out even routine activities. Confusion, disorientation, and profound memory problems can develop. Obvious motor abnormalities reflecting peripheral neuropathy may appear, such as ataxia, spastic leg weakness, generalized hyperflexia, and motor slowing (Coates, Stall *et al.*, 1987; Ho *et al.*, 1985; Navia & Price, 1986; Vishnubhakat, Kaplan, & Beresford, 1987). The progression and course of AIDS dementia is highly variable. Some patients deteriorate slowly over many months before they become globally impaired, while others may deteriorate dramatically in a period of several weeks.

In the late stages of AIDS dementia, computerized axial tomography (CAT or CT) scans have documented evidence of central and cortical atrophy with ventricular enlargement (Siegal *et al.*, 1987). Electroencephalogram (EEG) results reflect a mild, diffuse slowing, and lumbar puncture may reveal elevated protein or mononuclear pleocytosis (Ho *et al.*, 1987; Holland & Tross, 1985; Levy *et al.*, 1985; Navia & Price, 1986; Snider *et al.*, 1983; Wolcott, 1986b). Navia & Price (1986) indicate that the major neuropathological abnormalities are found in the white matter of subcortical brain structures and cortical gray matter evidences few changes. There is some evidence to suggest that brain areas responsible for language-related functions may be more selectively affected by HIV infection than other areas of the brain (Brouwers, Hobak, Squillace, Joffe, & Rubinow, 1987).

7.4. PSYCHOLOGICAL CONSEQUENCES OF ARC AND AIDS TO OTHERS

The psychological consequences described thus far in this chapter directly affect the person diagnosed with ARC or AIDS. However, the diagnosis also affects lovers, friends, family members, and the health care providers who care for AIDS patients while they live and as they die.

7.4.1. Effects on Spouses and Lovers

Spouses, spouse-equivalents, and lovers are simultaneously confronted with the terminal diagnosis of a loved one and inevitable worries about whether they, too, will become ill. With most other terminal diagnoses, relationship partners respond by drawing nearer to the diagnosed individual. Following an AIDS diagnosis, supportive and compassionate responses may be more strained since the lover is confronted with both the partner's deteriorating health and his or her own vulnerability. If the AIDS patient is a gay man with a male lover, there may be less recognition of the partner's needs and distress than if the patient were heterosexual and married. Partners, too, are often in need of mental health services as they attempt to cope with the future loss of their loved one and their own uncertainty about whether they may face the same illnesses.

7.4.2. Families

Families of AIDS patients face multiple stressors. In addition to coping with the eventual death of the AIDS patient, family members often must come to terms with their feelings about the patient's life-style, with stigma because a member of their family has AIDS, and with their own fears concerning the illness. Developing mental health resources to better assist these families not only will benefit the AIDS patient and the family members but also has broader social implications. Expanding available services to family members can be justified as cost-effective health care. The increasing numbers of AIDS-affected persons threaten to overwhelm our health care system, and growing numbers of patient beds are required for persons with AIDS. Inpatient care is also expensive and may have to be prolonged if a family feels unable or unwilling to assist in the home care of a patient too ill to resume independent living. Family interventions can enable the family to provide home care and support benefiting the patient and reducing the need for extended hospitalization or residential care.

7.4.3. Caregivers

Those who care for AIDS patients are affected by the stress of the health crisis. AIDS is a merciless killer and most patients die within 2 years of their AIDS diagnoses. Caregivers accustomed to curing their patients become taxed by their inability to provide substantive remedies to patients in the late stages of their disease. Often the tools of caregivers consist of little beyond reassurance, emotional support, and compassion. As a result, providers become frustrated by their inability to restore health to their AIDS patients. For those who have chosen to become involved primarily in working with AIDS patients, the toll of watching young people in the prime of life waste away takes a heavy emotional toll. Caregivers may also be ostracized by professional peers who are uncomfortable with the disease or with the life-styles of AIDS patients (Ottenberg, 1986). This can lead to the provider's becoming isolated from collegial contact and support.

Many health care providers fear contagion, even though a growing body of research indicates that health care workers are at little risk if standard body fluid precautions are followed. Reed, Wise, and Mann (1984) surveyed 267 nurses and found that 67% were anxious about catching AIDS from their patients. When over 1,000 health care workers were followed in a surveillance project after they had become exposed to HIV-infected blood through needlestick injuries and other accidental on-the-job exposures, only 0.5% subsequently seroconverted (Marcus *et al.*, 1987). Furthermore, 40% of those accidental exposures would not have occurred if the staff had followed recommended body fluid procedures. When blood samples from nurses caring for children with AIDS and ARC were examined for HIV antibodies, none were HIV-exposed, even though the nurses cared for these children daily—giving baths, feeding, caring for catheters, administering intravenous medications, handling blood and urine specimens, having contact with blood and secretions, and touching and comforting the children (Boland, Keresztes, Evans, Oleske, & Connor, 1987). Similarly, when a sample of dentists and surgeons who cared for HIV-affected patients were tested, none had antibodies to the HIV by Western blot analysis (Harper *et al.*, 1987).

In spite of this knowledge, there can be a gap between cognitive knowledge and personal attitudes (Reed *et al.*, 1984). In a survey of general practice physicians and pediatricians in New York, 48% of the general medical and 30% of the pediatric physicians reported moderate to major anxiety about acquiring AIDS from their patients (Link, Feingold, Charap, Freeman, & Shelov, 1987), and more than 25% of the physicians in the study believed a physician could ethically refuse to treat an AIDS-affected patient. A similar study conducted in California assessed health care workers' estimation of risk and anxiety from caring for persons with AIDS (Cooke & Koenig, 1987). Interestingly, significant differences were found between male and female medical house officers' estimation of risk; 84% of the men but only 48% of the women believed house officers were at risk if they cared for AIDS patients. More than 20% of the physicians reported they were "very anxious" about contracting AIDS from their patients, and 97% acknowledged that they worried about contracting AIDS at least occasionally. Twenty percent reported having nightmares about AIDS, and 18% of the physicians reported detecting symptoms in themselves that they erroneously interpreted as possible symptoms of AIDS (Cooke & Koenig, 1987). It is evident that health care providers are vulnerable to increased stress even as they meet their professional responsibilities to AIDS-affected patients.

Psychosocial Care Needs of Persons with AIDS

We do not see ourselves as victims. We will not be victimized.
We have the right to be treated with respect, dignity, compassion, and understanding.
We have the right to lead fulfilling, productive lives—
to live and die with compassion and dignity.
Mission statement of the National Association of People with AIDS

Persons diagnosed with frank AIDS are not a uniform group and do not have uniform needs. Some AIDS patients are first seen in the late stages of their illnesses when death is imminent. Others are seen much earlier, during a period of relatively good health or during an acute illness from which they will recover. Some AIDS patients are incapacitated by debilitating illness or impaired cognitive functioning. Others are alert, vigorous, and able to live independently and actively for months or even years. The emotional issues that confront an AIDS patient who is near death are very different from the issues relevant to the person with AIDS, who is in a prolonged remission. Because the health course associated with AIDS is not uniform and consistent, and because the same individual may experience worsenings and improvements in health, no single intervention strategy is relevant for all patients.

Persons with AIDS differ in their social and environmental support needs. Some patients have close, supportive social networks and are cared for by family members or relationship partners during times of illness. Others are homeless and have few supports and few resources. Access to psychosocial, economic, and social supports may differ across persons in the various current high-risk groups. In New York, for example, intravenous drug users with AIDS are predominantly poor and black or Hispanic, while gay men with AIDS are more often white, educated, and with above-average incomes. For chronic drug users, the AIDS diagnosis often compounds with preexisting social and economic stressors as well as the effects of long-term intravenous drug use (Lyons, Cossaboom, Graham, Honey, & Landesman, 1987).

Psychological and social interventions must take into account the heterogeneity of persons who are diagnosed with AIDS as well as the complex biopsychosocial characteristics of the disease. Some patients are able to adjust satisfactorily to the knowledge that they have AIDS; others require supportive psychotherapy interventions similar to those that are often used for most patients who face life-threatening illness. Still other clients require comprehensive intervention involving a number of interdisciplinary specialties. For these individuals, adequate service delivery may require liaisons among acute medical care hospitals and community housing, nursing, and hospice facilities; the provision of medical, psychological, social, legal, nursing, and pastoral care; and personal care, homemaker, meal, transportation, and financial support/ disability application assistance services (Crawford, 1987). An effective case management or multidisciplinary team approach can permit flexibility in service planning and coordination among the service providers from different specialities.

8.1. PSYCHOLOGICAL INTERVENTIONS

Psychological and social support interventions for persons with AIDS require a balance between assisting the client to live to the most active, productive, hopeful extent possible and, at the same time, to cope with the probability of a shortened life expectancy. As implied earlier, the health status and psychological adaptations of persons with AIDS are not static. During periods of relative health, issues involving activities and personal goals are important. The therapist's efforts can assist the client in maintaining hope and engaging in constructive life patterns. During other periods, coping with the prospect of death is a more salient issue. In the end stages of AIDS-related diseases, the therapist's role is often primarily supportive.

Although there is not yet a well-developed literature on psychosocial interventions that are helpful to persons with AIDS, the coping needs of patients with other life-threatening illnesses—in particular, cancer—have been examined and interventions to address those needs have been evaluated. Jay, Elliott, and Varni (1986), in a review of this literature, found that techniques emphasizing anxiety reduction (usually through relaxation training, hypnosis, or imagery/ meditation approaches), cognitive intervention to improve coping, social support provision, and goal-or activity-setting steps are useful for patients who are experiencing pain and who must cope with the threat of terminal illness. The same therapy elements have been recommended for counseling persons with AIDS who are in emotional distress (Abrams *et al.*, 1986). Many of the therapy techniques for HIV-seropositive persons discussed in Chapter 6 are therefore relevant for clients with AIDS or ARC illnesses. However, persons with AIDS-related illnesses not only face anxiety about their health but also have current health problems. Depending on the individual's stage and type of opportunistic illness, these can include: episodic or enduring pain; fatigue; fever; gastrointestinal dysfunction; wasting; physical disfigurement; sensory, motor or neurological limitations; and other impairments. Especially for individuals who are young and were formerly in good health, these symptoms are frightening and require difficult life adaptations. To the extent that therapists can assist clients in adapting to new physical challenges and living productively in spite of them, the client's quality of life can be maintained at the highest level possible.

Beyond social and emotional benefits, psychological adjustment may be related to length of survival. Effective coping is related to duration of survival following cancer diagnoses (Derogatis, Abeloff, & Melisaratos, 1979; Greer, Morris, & Perttingale, 1979) and to the probability of relapse within 1 year for certain types of cancer (Rogentine et al., 1979). Whether such relationships exist for AIDS and AIDS-related conditions has not been established. However, in addition to following established medical regimens, it cannot hurt—and may well benefit their health—for clients to be assisted in adopting active stress-coping skills, establishing feelings of control over behavior that can be controlled, and instituting healthful practices such as proper nutrition, exercise, sleep, and avoidance of intoxicants.

Considerable research indicates that social support buffers the impact of stressful life events (Cohen & Willis, 1985; Kessler & McLeod, 1985; Thoits, 1986; Turner, 1983). Since effective support often comes from others facing the same stressors (Gottlieb, 1978; Thoits, 1986) and because AIDS is frequently associated with feelings of isolation and diminished support (Pollak, Gharakhanian, *et al.*, 1987), persons with AIDS may derive particular benefit from involvement in support groups. Groups may be process-oriented, may be intended to help group members learn and implement coping skills, or may involve a combination of both. The key features of support groups include face-to-face interaction between the group members, an emphasis on personal and voluntary participation by each member, emotional support, and some identified similarity between members of the group (Katz & Bender, 1976). Because their needs, fears, and health outlook differ, it is probably advisable to offer separate groups for persons with AIDS, persons with ARC, those who are HIV-seropositive but asymptomatic, or other client populations.

The stress of an AIDS diagnosis is exacerbated when friends, family members, or health providers are not supportive (Coates, Stall, et al., 1987). Consequently, support groups are offered by many AIDS service programs. While no empirical literature has specifically evaluated the usefulness of social support groups for persons with AIDS, a considerable body of literature documents the benefits of support groups for persons suffering from other chronic or terminal illnesses. Close to 6 million patients with serious chronic diseases participate in such groups (Stokes, 1982). Social support has been shown to reduce psychological distress during periods of unusual stress (Billings & Moos, 1982; Kaplan, Robbins, & Martin, 1983) and to enhance recovery from serious illnesses (see Wallston, Alagna, DeVellis, & DeVellis, 1983, for a literature review). Two benefits of social support seem particularly applicable to persons with AIDS. One is that the client is able to talk freely about feelings in an environment where stigma is unlikely. Clients with AIDS may be relatively unable to talk about their fears, feelings, and coping efforts in other settings where ostracism and avoidance would result. This opportunity is perceived as helpful and desirable by persons experiencing life crises (see Dunkel-Schetter & Wortman, 1982). A second benefit is shared contact with others who are coping with a similar life crisis (Lehman, Ellard, & Wortman, 1986).

The literature on social support programs for cancer patients is applicable to persons with AIDS. Taylor, Falke, Shoptaw, and Lichtman (1986) described cancer in terms that apply equally well to AIDS. Both diagnoses introduce a stressor that requires continuing physical and psychological adjustments. Cancer patients and persons with AIDS both face the likelihood of deteriorating future health, as well as debilitating effects from their medical treatments. In addition, both diseases can be characterized by periods of remission between acute illnesses. During these interims, the person lives with uncertainty about further exacerbations and often worries about whether the next recurrence might be fatal (Dunkel-Schetter, 1984). The increased need for social support by cancer patients during those periods has been thoroughly documented (Bloom, 1982) and is very likely paralleled by persons with AIDS.

Many studies have demonstrated positive relationships between emotional support and a person's physical and psychological adjustment to cancer (Bloom, 1982; Funch & Metlin, 1982; Lichtman & Taylor, 1986; Taylor et al., 1985, 1986). Support from others at the time of a cancer diagnosis predicts lessened emotional distress and longer survival following diagnosis (Funch & Marshall, 1983; Vachon, 1979; Weisman & Worden, 1975), and support groups alleviate some of the psychosocial problems that arise following cancer (Maisiak, Cain, Yarbro, & Josof, 1981; Spiegel, Bloom & Yalom, 1981). They may play an even greater role in facilitating the adjustment and coping of AIDS patients primarily because of the paucity of other naturally occurring positive support opportunities for people with HIV conditions.

Death and dying are issues that confront an individual who has been diagnosed with AIDS. For many patients, fear of debilitation and death is the most critical, open emotional crisis following diagnosis and is raised immediately in counseling. Other persons choose not to discuss death and, instead, maintain their usual routine to the greatest degree possible until late stages of their illness. There is no doubt that most therapists and helping professionals are uncomfortable with discussions about death. However, patients can be assisted in dealing with these issues so they can shift their focus, as much as possible, to living with AIDS rather than dying from AIDS.

Kubler-Ross (1969) has identified common stages of death and dying, and mental health professionals working with HIV-affected persons should be familiar with these stages. Disbelief or denial, anger, depression, "bargaining," and acceptance are common psychological reactions to the threat of death. While these phenomena can be readily observed and described, there are no easy templates for counseling persons with a terminal diagnosis, and the issue of how best to work with AIDS patients confronting their own mortality has received little attention. Several writers, experienced in the care of dying patients who are depressed and suffering emotionally, have identified techniques useful for counseling persons coping with the possibility of death (Garfield, 1978; Kubler-Ross, 1969; Schofferman, 1986).

1. *Keep it simple.* Clinicians just beginning to work with the terminally ill or seeing their first few AIDS patients may find their own anxiety levels high. This inner discomfort can lead to over-talkativeness, the use of confusing language, jitteriness, stiff body posture, or failure to give the client adequate opportunity to talk or ask questions.
2. *Wait for questions.* Quiet is effective, allowing the client to express whatever feeling the diagnosis has produced, whether tears or anger. Be willing to wait for questions to arise.
3. *Find out what the diagnosis means to the client.* Misconceptions can be corrected. The client's interpretation and personal meanings attached to the diagnosis can be helpful in understanding how this particular diagnosis is affecting this particular person. In correcting misinformation and answering questions, there is opportunity to convey that you are knowledgeable and can help.
4. *Don't feel that you have to answer at one time every question that could arise.* People can absorb, recall, and mull only a limited amount of information at one time. There is no reason to feel that all the information needs to be provided at once. Start simply and give the information time to sink in before elaborating at the next visit.
5. *Don't argue with denial.* If the client wants or needs to deny after a certain point, respect his or her right to do so. Allow for denial and don't become overly confrontive. As the person's trust and confidence increases, communication may open.
6. *Check for understanding.* After you have provided information to the client, see what has been understood.
7. *Leave room for hope, but do not lie.* As Schofferman (1986) points out, one can always present a cup as being 10% full or 90% empty. Leave hope alive, while remaining truthful with the person.

8.2. OTHER CARE NEEDS FOLLOWING AIDS DIAGNOSIS

Clergy traditionally minister to families and patients facing serious illness and death. The roles of a pastor, priest, rabbi, or chaplain in ministering to persons with AIDS are important and are the same as ministering to persons with other illnesses. This may involve administering traditional rites and sacraments of faith; providing support and counseling for the patient as well as family, friends, and caregivers; and helping the patient reconcile unresolved spiritual issues. While some clergy and church denominations have long had ministries to the urban poor, homosexual, and nontraditional communities, ministering to persons with AIDS requires sensitivity to alternative life-styles and relationships and an ability to set aside judgments concerning aspects of the patient's behavior that may be in conflict with traditional church doctrine. Several resources are available to guide clergy who provide pastoral care to persons with AIDS (Murphy, 1986; South, undated).

Many of the problems faced by AIDS patients have both psychosocial and legal implications. In one study, approximately 50% of people with AIDS seen at a New York City hospital were found to be in need of some legal assistance (Gordon & Zuckerman, 1987). Attorneys are increasingly becoming included in multidisciplinary AIDS treatment teams in order to assist with sensitive aspects of legal planning. Legal services often needed include drafting powers of attorney, wills, and child custody and guardianship arrangements; providing assistance with housing, entitlements, and immigration status; and consulting on matters related to discrimination (Gordon & Zuckerman, 1987).

An issue with medical, psychological, and legal implications that usually arises after hospitalization involves reaching a decision regarding resuscitation status and the use of "heroic" measures if the patient's condition should worsen. At San Francisco General Hospital, patients admitted with a first episode of *Pneumocystis carinii* pneumonia are routinely counseled regarding the poor prognosis for patients with the disease who require intubation after an intensive care unit admission. This provides an early opportunity to discuss whether or not the patient wishes to be on full resuscitation status. Fewer than 10% of seriously ill patients choose to be on full code status (Fahrner, Clement, Kline, & Cohen, 1987).

8.3. ASSISTANCE WITH HOUSING AND HEALTH CARE RESOURCES

The AIDS epidemic has already begun to have a dramatic impact on hospitals. As the number of persons requiring medical care increases, alternatives to inpatient care will be increasingly needed. Green, Singer, and Winfield (1987) project that 12,831 hospital beds in the United States will be occupied by AIDS patients within the next 4 years. This exceeds the total number of beds that will be required for cancer patients or automobile accident victims. Furthermore, Green *et al.* (1987) note that the true impact goes well beyond these simple census figures, since AIDS patients often require added infection control precautions, nursing care, supplies, and more complex case management services.

While the costs of medical care for AIDS patients differ across the country, there is no question that acute care costs are high. A survey of Massachusetts hospitals over a 2-year period found that the inpatient cost of medical care averaged $42,517 per AIDS patient per year (Seage, Landers, Barry, Lamb, & Epstein, 1987). Comparable cost figures have been reported from New York (Drucker *et al.*, 1987). It is also clear that the costs of hospital care for AIDS patients are higher than for other patients. For example, Fanning, Harmon, Shepherd, Vellend, and Minnick (1987) found hospital costs of AIDS patients to be 31% greater than for patients with other illnesses. Over time, increasing numbers of AIDS-affected patients may not have third-party coverage for their hospital costs. Since uninsured patients typically can pay only about 5% of their hospital bills (Clark & McCallum, 1987), private hospitals will be increasingly unwilling to admit uninsured or minimally insured patients. The increasing demand for hospital beds by AIDS patients and the costs for care have fiscal implications for the globally budgeted public and nonprofit hospitals that provide most AIDS-patient care.

The hospital stay of patients with AIDS is sometimes prolonged unnecessarily. Substantial numbers of AIDS patients are homeless by the time of hospital admission or may not be accepted as patients by postacute care hospices or nursing homes, complicating discharge planning (Hurzeler, & Rawson, 1987). Surveys of hospitalized persons with AIDS have found that from 17 to 30% of patients are homeless or lack appropriate residential settings to which they can be discharged following an inpatient stay (Small, Laper, & Ricci, 1987; Wright, 1987). There are many reasons for this paucity of alternative living arrangements: ostracism by family, roommates, or lovers; evictions following the AIDS diagnosis; depletion of economic resources from illness expenses; and the reluctance of many nursing homes or hospices to admit AIDS patients (Wright, 1987). For some persons there may be difficulty returning to their previous home because family members or housemates are reluctant to accept them, while others may require transitional living arrangements before they are physically capable of returning to their homes. Some patients no longer need acute care, but do need a place in which they can live and die with dignity.

When patients who are no longer in need of acute care can be discharged to less care-intensive settings, the cost of care is substantially lower. Heseltine, Leedom, Hedderman, Ripper, and Sattler (1987) examined how a program of outpatient-based services affected inpatient resource utilization by persons with AIDS and AIDS-related illnesses. Over 2 years, there was a strong inverse relationship between the number of outpatient visits and inpatient lengths of stay, with a corresponding reduction in care costs for each patient served. Thus, a coordinated system for outpatient care not only reduces inpatient stays and medical care costs for persons with AIDS, but also is a flexible alternative for meeting the increasing needs for patient services.

Retaining patients in acute care facilities after they are medically ready to be discharged to less care-intensive settings is not cost-effective. In addition, unnecessarily protracted hospitalization can be detrimental to the patient's emotional well-being and disruptive of social supports. One solution to the problem of community care for AIDS patients who lack family or relationship supports is a system of transitional housing ranging from apartments for those capable of ambulatory self-care to hospice total care for the terminally ill, with hospitalization reserved for acute, intensive medical treatment (Feldman, Hummel, & Simmons, 1987). Such a coordinated program could allow for movement among alternative levels of care as they are required, would permit more efficient utilization of resources, and would enable AIDS patients to maintain the quality of their lives in a home environment as long as possible (Feldman et al., 1987; Perry, Rodriguez, Rotkiewicz, & Young, 1987). Transitional apartments, ambulatory day care, home-based support programs, and hospice care are being employed in various areas.

8.3.1. Transitional Apartments

Transitional apartments provide a lower-cost alternative to inpatient care for patients who are ambulatory, who are able to meet most of their own care needs, and who could be discharged from the inpatient setting if stable housing were available. When combined with regular personal assistance from trained paid or volunteer companions, a significant number of persons with AIDS who are not acutely ill could live successfully in the community. In New Jersey, such transitional self-help residences afforded a cost-effective and humane alternative for AIDS patients who no longer needed acute hospital care (Perry *et al.*, 1987). Unfortunately, the availability of transitional apartments is limited and insufficient to meet the need (Rodriguez & Jackson, 1987).

8.3.2. Ambulatory Day Care

Ambulatory day care programs are another alternative to residential care. In one such program, health-related services are provided daily to persons who are ambulatory and do not require inpatient care yet, owing to physical or mental impairment, need regular supportive services. The AIDS/ARC Medical Day Care Program in New Jersey provides medical, nursing, social, transportation, personal care, dietary, recreational, rehabilitative, drug counseling, and dental services for intravenous drug users diagnosed with AIDS (Rodriguez & Jackson, 1987), meeting patient needs in a cost-effective way that enable patients to remain in the community.

8.3.3. Home-Based Support Programs

Since severe illnesses often deplete financial resources, rent subsidies may be a feasible and low-cost way to enable people with AIDS to continue living in their own residences when they are capable of ambulatory self-care or when support is available to assist the person with personal care needs.

Several innovative programs that provide home-based support have enabled persons with AIDS to remain in their homes for as long as possible. These often combine daily social visitation, assistance with meals, home nursing care, and assistance with routine activities of daily living. When volunteer services are integrated into the comprehensive home health service program, many needs of persons with AIDS can be met in a humane and cost-efficient way. The AIDS Home Care and Hospice Program in San Francisco was the first such program in the country and has provided home care for more than 500 patients over a 3-year period (Martin, 1987).

An innovative program in New York City recruited volunteer methadone program clients to provide support for inner-city AIDS patients (Tenneriello *et al.*, 1987). In the program, 20 volunteers of socioeconomic background similar to that of the AIDS patients completed a 2-day training program and attended weekly volunteer support groups to receive professional supervision of their individual work. Over 6 months, the volunteers provided more than 1,000 hours of service to 30 persons with AIDS. In addition, they organized holiday celebrations for hospitalized patients. Tenneriello *et al.*, (1987) report that the program was successful in establishing a volunteer coalition from a diverse background; used methadone patients who are often stereotyped, discounted, and self-disparaging to help the AIDS-affected community while simultaneously increasing their own self-worth; and created a strong source of group support and bereavement consolation for survivors of deceased patients. Among the problems encountered were difficulties recruiting volunteers from a multiproblem, poorly functioning population of methadone clients, safeguarding against destructive experiences for the patients and the volunteers alike, providing adequate supervision for the volunteers, and securing funding for such a community-based program. Nonetheless, this peer-support approach is innovative and merits further evaluation.

8.3.4. Hospice Care

Many persons with advanced AIDS will require 24-hour care for weeks or months. Some are physically debilitated; others need a structured environment because of neurological deterioration. Hospice care provides special types of care for dying persons that are generally not available in traditional medical systems (DiTullio, 1986). Well-planned hospices are equipped to deal with the medical, social, and personal dilemmas that affect terminally ill persons. The availability of hospice care for AIDS patients has been limited. After an AIDS home care program was established in San Francisco, the need for 24-hour attendant care and supervision became evident and a hospice was opened specifically for terminally ill ARC and AIDS patients (Martin, 1987). The facility is staffed by licensed vocational nurses, attendants, volunteers, registered nurses, and social workers experienced in caring for the dying. Kutzen (1986) and Martin (1986) have written program overviews of AIDS hospice facilities developed in Louisiana and California, which describe the implementation of hospice care programs and offer guidance in staff training at existing hospices where AIDS-patient admissions are expected.

8.4. INTERVENTIONS FOR FAMILY MEMBERS
   AND SIGNIFICANT OTHERS

For every AIDS patient, an average of eight family members, relationship partners, and significant others are also directly affected by the patient's disease (Walker, 1987). Often, these are the individuals who care for the person with AIDS before or after hospitalizations. Families, relationship partners, or others who care for an AIDS patient may become stressed and burdened by the demands associated with this caregiving role. Families whose support needs are not met during the caretaking of a family member with AIDS report more depression, fatigue, guilt, anger, helplessness, and illness than families who felt their needs were met (Klein & Fletcher, 1987). The difficulties and unmet needs described by families who care for AIDS patients before their death include: inadequate social, legal, financial, or emotional supports; lack of knowledge about available community resource and assistance programs; limited understanding of how best to care for the patient at home; and difficulty communicating with health care professionals. Family members also have difficulty understanding and coping with changes in their relationship with the patient as death approaches (Klein & Fletcher, 1987). On the other hand, and with proper support, care for the dying may also have enduring beneficial effects for the caregiving family or friends. Several studies suggest that families who care for their terminally ill members find it difficult but also satisfying (Koocher, 1986; Martinson, Nesbit, & Kersey, 1984).

As discussed in Chapter 7, Friedland, Kahl, et al. (1987) found significant reductions in the frequency and closeness of interactions between family members and AIDS patients after their diagnosis. However, the same study found that when the family members became knowledgeable about the lack of transmission risk to household contacts who are not sexual partners of AIDS patients, normal personal interaction patterns were maintained (Friedland, Kahl, et al., 1987). This suggests the importance of clearly informing family members, other caretakers, and the patient that routine, close contact does not pose HIV transmission risk and that avoidance of regular household interactions is unwarranted. The only exception involves direct contact with blood or body secretions of patients who are seriously ill. However, family caretakers can be shown simple procedures, such as the use of gloves for changing dressings if that is necessary, that are protective but do not disrupt the social functioning of the household unit. It is essential that families or partners who care for loved ones with AIDS receive regular and adequate assistance from home health care and social service professionals.

In addition to providing information about AIDS and correcting misconceptions about household transmission, family members and relationship partners often require counseling assistance to cope with their own feelings and fears. Adapting to the loss of a loved one is one of life's most stressful events (Osterweis, Solomon, & Green, 1984; Videka-Sherman, 1982). While the patient is living, significant others may need an opportunity to discuss their anger, their conflicts concerning how the person became exposed to HIV infection, and their fears concerning loss of the patient. For some families, concern over the social stigma of a family member with AIDS may create significant additional stress. Following the AIDS patient's death, the mourning process may be complicated and intensified by the same factors (Koocher, 1986). Therapists who work with AIDS-affected families stress the importance of ongoing assistance from the time of diagnosis, through the caregiving period, and continuing after the death of the patient. The Ackerman Institute in New York City has long offered ongoing counseling support for family members, friends, spouses, and relationship partners of persons with AIDS (Walker, 1987). Others have noted the beneficial effects of social support and support groups on the emotional coping of survivors (Osterweis *et al.*, 1984; Parkes & Weiss, 1983; Rando, 1983), and grief recovery groups for the loved ones of patients who died of AIDS may be of particular benefit (Klein & Fletcher, 1987).

Difficult though it may be, bereavement is a universal experience, and families and loved ones coped with death for centuries before there were mental health professionals. Many will continue to do so. However, the possibility and then the reality of losing a loved one to this disease is a unique and particularly difficult stress. Developing service provisions to improve the adaptation of those who must cope with the loss of a loved one from AIDS is a sad but essential challenge in the health crisis.

8.5. INTERVENTIONS FOR CAREGIVERS

Earlier chapters identified professional issues that impact on caregivers. These include ethical issues, the need to remain abreast of developing information, sensitivity to and knowledge about alternative life-styles, comfort discussing sexual behavior, emotional burnout, and confronting fears of contagion. Caring for AIDS patients elicits strong psychological responses in care providers. In a study by Cooke and Koenig (1987), medical house staff who cared for large numbers of AIDS patients were less negative about patient care than those who had little personal experience. This suggests that some of the reticence in caring for persons with AIDS may be due to anticipatory anxiety that decreases with personal experience and patient contact. Yet Link *et al.* (1987) reported different findings. In their survey of house staff, physicians with increased AIDS patient contacts were more concerned about their personal health risk. In addition, when researchers surveyed medical and pediatric residents in four New York residency programs with large AIDS-patient populations, 30% indicated that concern about AIDS increased the stress of their residency to a moderate or extreme degree (Link *et al.*, 1987). While many professionals have responded to the crisis with sensitivity and compassion, these results suggest that providers may need assistance in handling stress and fear created by caring for AIDS patients.

Several programs have been developed to improve caregivers' professional development and continuing education. A collaborative effort by the New York City Department of Mental Health, the Memorial Sloan-Kettering Cancer Center, and the Gay Men's Health Crisis led to an AIDS mental health training program in New York City (Moynihan *et al.*, 1987). More than one thousand professionals from hospitals, community mental health centers, social service agencies, and chemical dependency programs have now participated in the program. An initial needs assessment revealed that presenting information about the medical and psychosocial aspects of AIDS was not sufficient to address issues relevant to these professionals. The substantive areas that the professionals identified as training needs included fears of contagion, homophobic prejudice, aversion to treating drug users, feelings of hopelessness and helplessness, emotional overload, working with the terminally ill, coping with the enormity and intensity of patient needs, and maintaining updated medical information. Five additional areas also addressed in the program included drug addiction, minority cultural issues, neuropsychological issues, and family and relationship therapy skills. Participation in the program did not significantly impact upon participants' factual knowledge because most were knowledgeable before the program began. After participating, however, 73% reported more optimism in helping persons with AIDS to cope with their illness, 75% reported greater empathy for persons with AIDS, more than 80% indicated they were more confident about their AIDS knowledge and more aware of the psychological and medical needs, and more than 60% felt better able to deal with the value and life-style differences encountered in working with persons with AIDS.

An innovative "Train the Trainer" program for mental health professionals was implemented in California to address the fears and misunderstandings related to AIDS-patient care. Seven-hundred-and-fifty key health care professionals participated in 2-day staff training programs based on experiential learning principles to convey information about AIDS. Creative teaching strategies, such as guided fantasy, role-play, and simulations, were used in place of more traditional didactic lectures to encourage group interactions and analysis of the sensitive issues implicated in fear of AIDS. Each of the 750 persons trained then conducted instructional programs for groups of 25 or more health care professionals from his or her home area. In those secondary sessions, an additional 18,750 people, including direct care personnel, support staff, and hospital administrators, were trained (Schietinger, Fitzhugh, McCarthy, & Morrison, 1987). Within a short period of time, this innovative approach allowed for information dissemination throughout the state's health care system.

Another broad-based professional education program was developed at the University of California, San Francisco (Mandel, Grade, et al., 1987). Five thousand health care professionals will attend seminars addressing HIV-related diseases as well as the psychosocial, legal, and ethical complexities of AIDS. The program emphasizes diagnosis, treatment, prevention, and health education and is intended to sensitize participants to issues affecting racial minorities, substance users, gay and bisexual men, transfusion recipients, women, and children.

Nurses also experience severe stress in caring for AIDS patients. Seidl and Goebel (1987) have described an intervention to reduce nurses' stress utilizing groups that met weekly for 6 months. In the first few months of the program, attitudes expressed by the nurses reflected hostility. AIDS patients were described as being more demanding than other patients. However, the nurses had difficulty handling patient demands, and their inability to restore AIDS patients to health raised feelings of ineffectiveness or of "not being a good nurse" (Seidel & Goebel, 1987). And as a result of caring for patients with a stigmatizing illness, the nurses felt themselves to be stigmatized by other hospital staff. These issues produced high levels of chronic stress. Seidel and Goebel (1987) reported that the process-oriented group intervention permitted nurses to express these concerns. The authors also reported that as nurses were able to identify and verbalize their frustrations, stress was reduced.

AIDS education and training for students in health-related careers can be incorporated into curricula before the students are placed in direct contact with persons who have HIV-related conditions. Such programs seem likely to benefit students and patients equally. At the University of California, San Francisco, a special course was developed for medical, nursing, and pharmacy students (Bartnof, 1987). The 13-hour course includes both lectures and panel discussions. The lectures review AIDS epidemiology, treatment of AIDS-related illnesses, clinical manifestations of AIDS, infection control, legal issues, public policy, and ethics. The panels include persons with AIDS and ARC as well as representatives from community AIDS health care systems. Students are assessed on their knowledge and attitudes before and after completing the course and show decreased AIDS-related fears and increased knowledge about HIV after completing the course. Such courses can serve an important educational function, which leads to increased professional knowledge and comfort about AIDS and ultimately improves the quality of AIDS-patient care.

Effective Help-Providing
Knowledge, Sensitivities, and Ethics

AIDS is a unique illness, the most frightening and serious of the sexually transmitted diseases. Since it appeared, AIDS has eclipsed much of the attention once given to such treatable "traditional" sexually transmitted diseases as syphilis, gonorrhea, and chlamydia, and even such non-curable ones as genital herpes. As discussed earlier, widespread fears that AIDS can be contracted through casual social contact remain, even though well-controlled studies repeatedly disconfirm any basis for this fear. The long latency between viral exposure and any disease onset and the fact that most HIV carriers appear visibly healthy also contribute to the uniqueness of the disease. Finally, because of its association with homosexuality, drug use, and sexual behavior, AIDS elicits stigmatizing and prejudicial attitudes with respect to the perceived life-styles of its victims.

Across a set of studies, the authors have examined attitudes toward persons with AIDS. In an initial study (St. Lawrence *et al.*, in press), 300 college students were presented with a 500-word vignette describing an individual named "Mark." The vignette described Mark as a hardwork-ing, athletic, active person with many hobbies and friends. In the sce-nario, it was reported that Mark became ill, had a series of recurrent infections, consulted his physician, and, after tests were performed, was told that he had a life-threatening illness. The vignette said that Mark became progressively more withdrawn and depressed, that his family and friends visited him less frequently because they were uncomfortable with the fact that he was probably dying, and that even Mark's long-standing romantic partner eventually left him.

The vignettes given to subjects were identical except for a manipulation of two words: Mark's illness was identified as either AIDS or leukemia, and the name of Mark's romantic partner was listed as either Roberta or Robert. After reading one of the four randomly assigned vignettes (homosexual with AIDS, heterosexual with AIDS, homosexual with leukemia, or heterosexual with leukemia), subjects completed objective, Likert-format measures assessing their attitudes toward Mark and their willingness to interact socially with him in a variety of everyday situations.

Results of the study revealed the presence of clear and distinctive differences in attitude toward Mark, depending on whether he was reported to have AIDS or leukemia and whether he was identified as heterosexual or homosexual. When Mark was said to have AIDS, subjects described him as being much more responsible for, and deserving of, his illness than when he was depicted as a leukemia patient; less deserving of sympathy; more deserving to die; and more dangerous, deserving of quarantine, and deserving to lose his job. If he did die, subjects reported that the death of the AIDS patient would represent a less important loss to the world than the death of the identically described leukemia patient. Further, across all social interactions included in the measure, such as having a simple conversation, working in the same office, or living in the same apartment building, subjects were markedly less willing to interact with the AIDS patient. Interestingly, a very similar pattern of prejudicial attitudes and unwillingness to interact was found when differences due only to the sexual preference manipulation in the vignette were examined. Regardless of their illnesses, patients labeled as homosexual were evaluated with much harsher attitudes than identically described heterosexual patients (St. Lawrence *et al.*, in press).

In subsequent studies, the same experimental paradigm was employed to experimentally assess the attitudes toward AIDS patients of medical students (Kelly, St. Lawrence, Smith, Hood, & Cook, 1987a), nurses (Kelly, St. Lawrence, Hood, Smith, & Cook, in press), and a sample of randomly selected physicians practicing in three large cities with moderate prevalence of AIDS (Kelly, St. Lawrence, Smith, Hood, &

Cook, 1987b). While the specific results varied slightly across samples, each of these investigations found that even health care professionals expressed much less willingness to interact in any way with a person described as having AIDS than with a person said to have leukemia. AIDS patients were consistently judged to be more deserving of their illness, less deserving of sympathy, and otherwise evaluated more harshly than leukemia patients. Medical students, for example, reported that the AIDS patient should more strongly consider suicide than the identically described leukemia patient.

Although these studies employed relatively small samples and did not examine whether attitudes might become less prejudicial as a result of increased contact with AIDS patients, the findings are consistent with large-scale public opinion polls that confirm the prevalence of harsh, judgmental, and fearful attitudes concerning persons with AIDS (Fisher, 1986; Newsweek, 1985; Siegel, 1986). During the past several years, proposals have been advanced to tattoo or quarantine persons with AIDS and HIV infection, children with AIDS have been kept from attending school, and persons with AIDS have been denied health care, housing, and employment owing to unwarranted fears of casual transmission (Brown, 1987; Matthews & Neslund, 1987; Young, 1986). Reported street violence directed against persons simply suspected of being gay has doubled to tripled in some large cities since the beginning of the AIDS health crisis (National Gay and Lesbian Task Force, 1987). Such phenomena indicate that much of the public and, unfortunately, many health care professionals are substantially uninformed about how AIDS can be transmitted. Moreover, this also suggests that at least some of the stigma associated with AIDS reflects not just fear of the disease but also disdain and prejudice toward its victims. AIDS is not viewed with impartiality by most people.

Because AIDS is a unique disease, special knowledge and sensitivities are required of professionals who work with persons affected by AIDS and certain ethical concerns assume increased importance. In this chapter, we will consider some of these issues.

9.1. KNOWLEDGEABLE CAREGIVING

Counseling persons who are either at risk for HIV infection or already exposed to the virus requires that a professional be knowledgeable about human sexuality, homosexual and heterosexual practices that carry high or low risk for HIV transmission between partners, intravenous drug use, and other risk-related behaviors. In addition, effective psychosocial interventions require the professional to be knowledgeable about life-style issues relevant for the individual being counseled. Since most current AIDS patients, HIV-infected persons, and AIDS at-risk persons are homosexual or bisexual males, it is essential that the caregiver be familiar with life-style, relationships, community support, and stressors that affect gay men. Members of other groups at risk for AIDS, including intravenous drug users, prostitutes, and heterosexuals with multiple partners, often have backgrounds quite different from those of the professionals who care for them. Only by becoming knowledgeable about the life-styles of persons affected by AIDS can professionals provide effective assistance.

Unfortunately, the background knowledge and competencies required to skillfully assist persons with HIV diseases or persons at risk for these disease are rarely taught in most professional training programs. Medical, nursing, social work, psychology, and counseling personnel have often had only minimal training in human sexuality and may be quite unfamiliar with sexual practices relevant to HIV transmission and prevention. It is rare for training programs to teach helping profession students to deal with the behavior and the problems encountered by gay persons, drug users, or the sexually promiscuous. And, while black and Hispanic persons account for a disproportionately large number of AIDS cases, minority mental health and public health issues often receive only cursory attention in traditional professional training programs. It is perhaps for these reasons that the most active AIDS-prevention campaigns and service programs for persons with AIDS have either originated in the gay community itself or been developed by public health organizations in close cooperation with gay community leaders. However, as the magnitude of the health crisis expands, professionals who have never been involved with AIDS-affected persons will develop interests in the area or will find themselves in the position of counseling patients with AIDS or individuals at risk for HIV infection.

9.1.1. Knowledge of Sexual Behavior

AIDS is primarily a sexually transmitted disease. But, as discussed in Chapter 2, not all sexual practices carry equal risk for permitting HIV transmission. In order to help at-risk persons reduce their exposure risk and in order to effectively counsel HIV-exposed persons, a caregiver must become knowledgeable about sexual behavior and the transmission risks associated with various sexual activities. The topic of risk levels was discussed in Chapter 2. However, professionals who are not experienced in taking a sexual history or assessing sexual behavior may wish to consult a more detailed resource (see Gremminger, 1983; Pomeroy, Flax, & Wheeler, 1982). It is particularly important that caregivers be aware of the diversity of sexual activities that occur between both heterosexual and homosexual partners. It is also important that "uniformity myths" concerning sexual behavior be avoided. Such activities as oral intercourse, anal intercourse, and oral–anal contact are not uncommon between heterosexual partners (Padian *et al.*, 1987), and a significant proportion of primarily heterosexual adult males have engaged in at least some homosexual activities (Gadpaille, 1985). The notion that persons can be dichotomously categorized as either homosexual or heterosexual, or that knowledge of a person's primary sexual preference predicts the specific sexual activities in which he or she engages, is often incorrect and may lead to incorrect assumptions and counseling about risk.

9.1.2. Knowledge about AIDS and HIV Infection

AIDS has been studied for only a brief period of time but, because research developments have occurred quickly, "new" information also becomes out-of-date and insufficient very rapidly. There are few areas where effective intervention requires that a professional remain abreast of such complex and rapidly changing medical, behavioral, and epidemiological information. This can be most clearly seen with respect to risk and prevention. Just a few years ago, it was widely accepted that HIV-infection risk was largely confined to homosexual males who lived in large cities, had extraordinarily large numbers of sexual contacts, and primarily engaged in receptive anal intercourse with those partners. As a result of the expanding nature of the health epidemic and better research methods, most of these assumptions are no longer accurate. Today, HIV infection is prevalent in all states and is not confined to large cities. Only a few sexual contacts are needed for gay men to encounter an HIV-infected partner, and it is known that sexual activities other than receptive anal intercourse can result in HIV transmission. Moreover, as HIV infection becomes more prevalent in the heterosexual community, heterosexually active persons with no homosexual practice background are at increased risk for infection. Prevention counseling must not only take into account these epidemiological changes but must also anticipate them.

In addition to prevention and changing risk-group trends, professionals who provide psychological and social services should be familiar with basic medical and health course aspects of HIV-infection diseases. In particular, it is important that professionals understand the differences between asymptomatic HIV infection, the various disease conditions associated with immunoinsufficiency, and symptoms of AIDS itself. Nonphysician professionals will not be called upon to diagnose patients but should be sufficiently familiar with health symptoms of HIV-related illnesses that they can accurately answer basic questions asked by patients, gauge when medical consultation is needed, and counsel individuals on HIV risk or transmission reduction. There are now several excellent resources and texts that review basic medical aspects of AIDS and HIV infection (DeVita *et al.*, 1985; Ebbesen *et al.*, 1984; Staquet *et al.*, 1986).

As we discussed in Chapter 7, persons with the more serious HIV-infection diseases, especially AIDS, often have multiple needs that require interdisciplinary professional attention. In addition to medical treatment, AIDS patients frequently require psychological, social, spiritual, financial, and home health care assistance. Both AIDS patients and some persons with serious HIV disorders other than AIDS have support and community living assistance needs that can also be met by nonprofessional caregivers. In order for interdisciplinary professional and nonprofessional programs to be maximally effective, it is important that all individuals involved in caregiving roles to AIDS patients be knowledgeable not only of the medical aspects of the syndrome but also of the social, psychological, and other stresses faced by persons with AIDS.

9.1.3. Knowledge of Life-Style Issues

Most current AIDS patients are individuals who were stigmatized even before the health crisis began, whether by virtue of their sexual preference, drug use, or multiple sexual partner activities. While the life-style profile of AIDS patients may gradually shift as the epidemiology of the disease changes, the majority of AIDS patients will continue for some years to be gay or bisexual males, intravenous drug users, and their direct or indirect sexual partners. Racial minority groups are projected to continue to account for a disproportionately high number of AIDS cases (Gerald *et al.*, 1987).

Although it is not necessary for professionals to be members of the same groups they assist, an extensive body of literature indicates that effective social and psychological intervention can be accomplished only when clients perceive the care provider to be understanding of their life-style, nonjudgmental, and genuinely concerned about their well-being (Truax *et al.*, 1966; Truax & Mitchell, 1971). To the extent that profession-als are not knowledgeable about life-style issues affecting persons with AIDS, or to the extent that the professional is uncomfortable with the client's life-style, barriers to care exist. There are several areas where knowledgeability is especially important.

9.1.3.1. Knowledge of Available Community Resources

Many large cities now have community programs for persons with AIDS, including peer support groups for AIDS patients, for those who are asymptomatic but HIV-positive, and for relatives or friends of per-sons with AIDS. Volunteer-staffed visitation and "buddy" programs that provide assistance in community living, personal care home and hospice facilities, and ministries for persons with AIDS are also present in many areas. Often developed by organizations in the gay community, these services are generally available to AIDS patients regardless of their sex-ual preference.

9.1.3.2. Knowledge of Relationship Supports

There is great diversity in the relationship supports available to per-sons with AIDS, especially patients who are homosexual. Some gay men enjoy close, open relationships with their families; others are much more "closeted." A common and most difficult task faces the homosexual AIDS patient who must explain not only his illness but also his sexual preference to family members unaware of either. Under these circum-stances, the probability of strained relationships and ostracism is, unfor-tunately, great. Counseling assistance to cope with this strain is often needed for the patient and for family members alike.

Care providers should also be knowledgeable about significant relationships that may exist between the patient and others, especially committed or "spouse-equivalent" relationships. The needs and fears of persons who have committed relationships with the AIDS or AIDS-affected patients often go unrecognized by care providers, probably because these relationships are not socially sanctioned in an identifiable, traditional sense. Just as the psychological needs of spouses often require attention when the patient is an ill heterosexual, professionals who provide care to homosexual AIDS patients should be sensitive to the potential presence and needs of "significant others" in the life of the patient.

Feelings of isolation, loneliness, and "contamination" are common in patients with AIDS or with other HIV-infection illnesses, and in persons who are seropositive to HIV. Not surprisingly, a substantial number of patients become withdrawn and depressed in addition to anxious and fearful about their health status. As discussed in Chapter 7, psychosocial interventions for persons affected by AIDS often entail helping the individual become involved with socially supportive individuals and organizations. In order to do so, the care provider must be knowledgeable about resources that are available in the community. For example, some gay persons with HIV illnesses wish to become involved in religious activities but feel alienated from traditional churches by virtue of their sexual preference or their illness. In such cases, it is useful for the care provider to know which traditional churches have programs sensitive to the needs of persons with AIDS and to be aware of churches and groups that specifically serve homosexual individuals. Examples are the Metropolitan Community Church, a denomination that serves the gay and lesbian community in many cities, and organizations such as Dignity and Integrity, composed primarily of gay Catholics and Episcopalians. Almost all such groups have formal or informal support programs for people affected by AIDS. In similar fashion, gay community organizations, health clinics that treat large numbers of AIDS patients, and state or regional AIDS task forces are often useful sources of information about social support services that are available in a given city. Professionals who provide psychosocial intervention to persons with AIDS should become knowledgeable about such community social support resources and should establish cooperative relationships with them.

Because the majority of current American AIDS patients are homosexual, most community service programs for persons with AIDS were initiated by gay community organizations. This is probably because persons in the gay community, affected most harshly by AIDS, saw the need to develop social service programs that "mainstream" health organizations were reluctant to undertake. For nonhomosexual AIDS patients, the association of AIDS services with identified gay community organizations can be a source of potential discomfort. Ideally as AIDS becomes more widely perceived as an illness unrelated to sexual preference *per se*, there will also be increased recognition of the need for compassionate, high-quality community, social, and health care services for all persons affected by AIDS, regardless of how they become exposed to HIV infection.

9.2. ETHICAL ISSUES

Psychosocial interventions for persons with AIDS or HIV infection raise special ethical issues. One set of issues involves confidentiality. While therapeutic interventions always require sensitivity toward client rights to privacy, the stigma associated with AIDS and the stigma that is associated with merely being perceived as at risk for AIDS mandates extraordinary diligence in maintaining confidentiality. Confidentiality safeguards include handling any client records or notes with great care to prevent unauthorized persons from learning their content; utilizing coded records without names or traceable personal identifiers when there is the possibility of unauthorized entry to records or record-keeping areas; seeing clients in locations or settings where simple client presence in the setting would not expose the individual to potential embarrassment or stigma; and otherwise protecting the individual's privacy. Special confidentiality safeguards are also warranted in the conduct of AIDS research (Bayer , Levine, & Murray, 1984).

A difficult ethical problem occurs when an individual known to be HIV-infected continues to engage in activities that can result in transmission of the virus to others. Fortunately, with proper counseling, most persons who learn they are HIV-seropositive following voluntary testing appear to behave in a responsible manner and do not engage in activities that pose transmission risk to others (Coates, Morin, & McKusick, 1987; Farthing *et al.*, 1987) However, there will be some cases in which persons who know they are HIV-infected continue to engage in high-risk sexual practices, needle sharing, or even prostitution. It is very likely that public health authorities will increasingly seek and use legal means to deal with HIV-infected individuals who knowingly engage in activities that pose clear risk to others. The questions of whether "failure to warn" statutes, which require mental health professionals to abridge usual confidentiality standards and to alert known potential victims of an individual's life-threatening behavior, apply to AIDS transmission has not yet been legally addressed. This ethical question can arise when an individual knows he or she is HIV-infected, when the individual's spouse or relationship partner is unaware of that HIV status, and when high-risk activities occur between them. If counseling the HIV-infected partner to alter risk practices is ineffective, a therapist might have to choose between breaching the client's confidentiality in an attempt to protect the partner—and thereby risking litigation—and maintaining confidentiality and placing the partner at risk (Bayer, Levine, & Wolf, 1987; Matthews & Neslund, 1987; Mills, Wofsy, & Mills, 1986). Fortunately, this ethical dilemma is not likely to occur frequently. As discussed earlier, HIV transmission primarily occurs between partners who do not know they are infected. Large-scale education and behavior-change efforts that encourage all at-risk individuals to consistently protect themselves and their partners from possible HIV exposure represent, in general, the most effective, realistic, and ethical broad-scale prevention approach (Solomon, in press).

AIDS attracts intense public notice, and there are many areas of public misunderstanding about the syndrome, especially unreasonable fears pertaining to casual transmission. When the public is alarmed and frightened, incorrect information or opinions that are not well grounded in fact can exacerbate hysteria, foster misinformation, and adversely affect the quality of life and civil liberties of persons with AIDS. As a result of tabloid stories and public opinions offered by irresponsible or unknowledgeable individuals, many people still believe that HIV infection can be transmitted by mosquitoes or cockroaches, that exposure can occur as a result of sharing the same workplace, or that food preparers can transmit the virus to persons who dine in the restaurants where they work. No data support any of these propositions. Nonetheless, because the public is frightened about AIDS, incorrect statements—especially if offered by a professional—are apt to be believed and can obscure the public's understanding of genuine, important risk behaviors. This implies an ethical responsibility for professionals to discuss AIDS in a highly accurate manner, to ensure that public statements are well supported by objective, scientific data, and to be aware that personal views are likely to be construed as factual by the public and by other professionals who are less knowledgeable about AIDS. By conveying information responsibly and by personally modeling constructive sensitivities, professionals are in a position to foster more accurate and compassionate responses by others.

9.2.1. Other Ethical Considerations

The AIDS crisis also raises other more specific ethical questions. Some directly confront the individual professional who treats persons with AIDS and HIV illnesses. Others are questions that will require careful ethical deliberation by those who plan public health policy.

9.2.1.1. Confidentiality with Respect to Disclosures Concerning Health Status

Providers of health care and social/psychological services may be requested to provide information concerning patients to third parties, including insurance companies, employers or their agents, or clinic patient record departments. The nature of the information that is disclosed may carry significant ramifications to the client or the patient. For example, if an individual were being counseled concerning HIV-antibody test results, and if that information became known, the individual's future health and life insurability would be in jeopardy and the individual could encounter discrimination with respect to employment and housing. Insurance companies have argued that failure to make HIV-antibody status known, or efforts to withhold such information from them, will result in heavy financial burdens for insurers (Myers, 1987). Organizations concerned with civil liberties point out that even confirmed HIV-antibody-positive status does not necessarily predict illness, that confidentiality safeguards concerning the sharing of this information about clients are inadequate, and that fear of losing insurability, employment, and other benefits or rights are realistic (Schatz, 1987; Schulman, Karp, & Nickens, 1987; Tillett, 1987). Several states and the District of Columbia prohibit insurance companies from denying life or health insurance to otherwise healthy persons who test positive for HIV antibodies, but most states do not afford such protections to those who are HIV-positive (*Hospitals*, 1986).

It is clearly an ethical responsibility of professionals to discuss with clients, in advance, what kinds of information will be maintained in records, what information might become released to insurers or others if health claims are filed, policies concerning client authorization to release information, whether there are requirements to report health conditions related to HIV infection, and protections to ensure record confidentiality. Because clients are often unaware of the potential ramifications of information that is released to third parties, professionals have an obligation to discuss these issues carefully with clients and to exercise great prudence with respect to any disclosures.

9.2.1.2. Sexuality after Learning about Positive HIV Status

As increasing numbers of persons seek HIV-antibody testing, an increasing number of persons will learn that they are seropositive to the virus and probably able to transmit it to others. An important ethical question involves how they should be counseled about their future sexual behavior.

It has been suggested that persons who learn they are HIV-antibody-positive should refrain from all sexual activity. Some states have passed, and others are considering passage of, laws to make the intentional transmission of HIV to others a criminal offense. Such legislation would be extremely difficult to enforce on a practical basis and, short of draconian invasions of privacy, sexual activities that occur between consenting adults are impossible to monitor or regulate. Available data also suggest that most persons who learn they are HIV-antibody-positive following voluntary testing attempt to modify their sexual behavior practices in ways to protect others (Coates, Morin, & McKusick, 1987; Farthing *et al.*, 1987).

The advice that should be given to persons with HIV antibodies or illness concerning future sexual activities should be both practical and ethical. On one hand, refraining from all sexual activity ensures the protection of others and also ensures that the HIV-positive individual will not be reexposed to the virus. On a practical basis, however, it is questionable whether most persons with a history of sexual activity will choose to become permanently celibate. From an ethical perspective, it seems essential to advise persons who know they are HIV-seropositive to make potential sexual partners aware of their HIV status and then to diligently adhere to sexual practices that pose the lowest risk for virus transmission (U.S. Department of Health and Human Services, 1986a).

9.2.1.3. Informed Consent and Decision Making
with Respect to Treatment

A significant proportion of persons with AIDS eventually develop neurological diseases that interfere with their cognitive functioning. In some cases, neurological symptoms are mild and nondebilitating. In other instances, the patient exhibits evidence of gross dementia and becomes unable to think or communicate coherently (Herman, 1986; Wolcott, 1986a). Under these circumstances, the patient is often unable to provide informed consent or participate in treatment decisions, including decisions about life-support maintenance at end stages of the disease.

It is desirable for professionals to solicit input concerning treatment and health care decisions, and to obtain consent, from a patient with AIDS who is showing some cognitive deterioration while the patient is still able to provide it. Such questioning requires extraordinary sensitivity and skill since , if undertaken insensitively, it can trigger increased feelings of despair and hopelessness. Because informed consent and decision making concerning the possible later use of experimental medical regimens, community placement and living arrangements, wills, and wishes concerning the use of life-support and resuscitation procedures involve legal issues, consultation with attorneys familiar with health care ethics and law is often necessary. In addition, it is important for health care professionals to obtain information from the AIDS patient about who should assist in decision making if the patient becomes unable to do so. In the event that the patient designates an individual without clear legal standing, such as a nonspouse lover, as a decision-making representative, legal consultation may also be necessary.

9.2.1.4. Mandatory HIV Antibody Testing

Most public health agencies, including the United States Public Health Service, recommend that confidential HIV-antibody testing be made widely available and recommend that individuals who suspect they are HIV-exposed seek voluntary testing (U.S. Department of Health and Human Services, 1986a). However, several states and federal agencies have enacted laws or requirements for mandatory HIV testing. Military personnel and immigrants are now required to submit to HIV-antibody testing, and laws have been introduced in various states to require HIV testing of persons applying for marriage licenses, prostitutes, prisoners, hospital patients, medical personnel, food service workers, teachers, schoolchildren, and various other groups. In coming years, mandatory testing statutes will no doubt be introduced and passed in legislatures at an increasing rate. Some of these laws stipulate that persons who test positive for HIV antibodies be denied employment and have their names registered in health authority files (Kaufman, Vergeront, & Frisby, 1987; Merritt, Rowe, & Ryan, 1987).

Proposals for mandatory HIV-antibody testing carry major public health policy ramifications and raise serous ethical concerns. Proposals for mandatory HIV testing of persons in most employment groups (such as food handlers, teachers, medical personnel, or cosmetologists) are unwarranted because AIDS and HIV infection have never been transmitted through their employment. While public fears concerning casual contagion exist, there is no scientific basic for fears that AIDS can be contracted in the workplace, office, or classroom (Friedland *et al.,* 1986; U.S. Department of Health and Human Services, 1986a). Legislation that is based on public misconceptions rather than on scientific data is imprudent, unnecessary, and dangerous.

In other cases, cost efficiency may argue against widescale mandatory HIV testing. Rather than test all patients entering hospitals in order to determine their HIV-antibody status and thereby determine for which patients body fluid precautions should be taken, it might be more effective, as well as safer and less costly, for medical personnel to simply upgrade the level of body fluid precaution taken with all patients. Mandatory HIV-antibody testing of couples seeking to marry may also represent a cost-inefficient prevention strategy. In most areas of the country, the prevalence of HIV infection among couples planning marriage is still likely to be exceedingly low (Brundage *et al.,* 1987; Schorr *et al.,* 1985). When the base rate prevalence of HIV infection in a given population is very low, the cost of mandatory testing becomes exceedingly high in relation to the number of HIV-infected persons who will be detected. One estimate indicates that if all American prisoners, immigration applicants, and couples applying for marriage licenses are screened for HIV antibodies, the cost per HIV-positive person detected will be about $10,000 (*The Economist,* 1987). A more viable, economic approach may be to recommend that couples who plan marriage, who suspect that they may be HIV-exposed, or who are concerned about AIDS, obtain confidential voluntary testing or follow safer sex precautions.

Even with increased funding for AIDS prevention, cost benefit relationships of various prevention approaches must be taken into account.

Wide-scale mandatory HIV-antibody testing is expensive, requires the use of costly repeated confirmatory tests other than the inexpensive ELISA in order to rule out false positives, and necessitates elaborate staffing arrangements to provide follow-up and counseling (*The Economist*, 1987). Proposals to trace the sexual contacts of HIV-positive persons have been advanced (see Merritt *et al.*, 1987), but such approaches would prove even more expensive and infeasible given the number of people who are HIV-exposed and the great probability of inaccurate or noncandid reports about past sexual contacts of the HIV-infected person. To the extent that federal, state, or local AIDS-prevention funds are diverted to support cost-ineffective mandatory testing programs, the funds available for more cost-efficient educational and prevention programs, as well as urgently needed biomedical research, are reduced. In essence, the key public health policy question is whether one should attempt to "find" and then attempt to monitor the private conduct of all persons who are HIV-exposed, clearly an impossible task, or whether one should instead educate and counsel the much larger proportion of the population that is not yet HIV-exposed in ways to protect themselves.

All proposals for involuntary HIV-antibody testing raise substantial issues concerning confidentiality, rights to privacy, and potential loss of civil liberties (Matthews & Neslund, 1987; Miller *et al.*, 1987). There is precedent for reporting communicable disease. Public health authorities have for many years monitored the incidence of certain diseases such as tuberculosis, typhoid, certain sexually transmitted diseases, and other contagious illnesses. However, these diseases differ from HIV infection because they are contagious through casual contact or are treatable. In addition, the presence of harsh attitude judgments toward AIDS risk-group members and people with AIDS (St. Lawrence *et al.*, in press) and widespread public misunderstanding about transmission of the disease suggest the strong potential for discrimination and ostracism. A Justice Department opinion that persons with AIDS can be fired from their employment with impunity if co-workers fear them, even when there is no legitimate medical basis for co-workers' fear of contagion, has done little to reassure those who are concerned about the civil liberties of persons affected by AIDS (Joseph, 1986).

When HIV testing is involuntary and carries the potential for breaches of confidentiality, loss of civil liberties, and invasion of privacy, it is likely that many persons who suspect they are HIV-exposed will evade health authorities. To the extent that populations at the greatest risk for becoming exposed to HIV infection and transmitting it to others have reason to distrust public health agencies, fear the social and civil liberties consequences of mandatory HIV testing, and become estranged from health care/public health systems, AIDS-prevention efforts will be hindered (Hopkins, 1987b). The groups at greatest current risk for AIDS —gay and bisexual men, intravenous drug users, the urban poor, and heterosexuals with multiple partners or with partners who are likely to HIV-infected—are difficult to reach in public health campaigns and the behaviors that create risk generally occur in private where they are undetectable. As a result, effective prevention efforts require voluntary, cooperative, trusting, and nonadversarial relationships between health authorities and people at risk for AIDS. If these relationships become eroded and if at-risk persons become unwilling to trust or utilize HIV testing, counseling, and health care resources, the spread of AIDS could accelerate even more quickly.

9.2.1.5. Costs of Health Care

In areas with the largest number of AIDS cases, the costs of patient care are creating heavy financial burdens for many nonprofit hospitals (Barnes, 1986; Brown *et al.*, 1987; *Nature*, 1987). Especially in cities such as New York, San Francisco, and Houston, community clinics and municipal public health agencies with limited budgets have had difficulty meeting the care needs of thousands of persons with AIDS and other HIV illnesses. As the number of AIDS patients increases, the resources of "high-incidence" cities will be further strained, and cities not yet heavily affected by AIDS will encounter similar difficulties. It is estimated that the medical care of patients will cost between $8 and $16 billion by 1991 (Barnes, 1986), although some projections are even higher.

AIDS is costly because persons with it develop frequent and recurring serious illnesses, often require multiple hospitalizations, and have substantial support and care needs between hospital admissions. Because a large proportion of individuals with HIV illnesses are unemployed and uninsured when their conditions become diagnosed, they often lack third-party health insurance and quickly become indigent. Medicaid funds cover some health care expenses of indigent persons with AIDS and related illnesses, and those who are disabled as a result of AIDS often qualify for modest disability income. However, these sources are insufficient to pay the costs of health care. In addition, promising new medications for the management of certain illnesses in immunocompromised patients are often expensive and are not always covered by third-party sources.

As the health crisis expands, there will be a need for greatly increased funding of health care services for persons with HIV illnesses. A variety of proposals for the better funding of AIDS patient care are under consideration and include increased Medicaid allocations, the establishment of specially "earmarked" federal AIDS funds that could be dispensed to states, and grant assistance to states, municipalities, or health organizations (*Congressional Quarterly*, 1987). Such efforts are clearly needed. Also needed are alternative health care service delivery systems for persons affected by AIDS. Cities with the largest number of AIDS patients for the longest time have moved toward comprehensive, community-based services integrating brief hospitalizations, when necessary, in AIDS specialty units with frequent outpatient follow-up; intensive, interdisciplinary home-based health and nursing care; assistance in meeting daily living needs; and hospice care for those terminally ill (Heseltine *et al.*, 1987; Wolfred, Dunne, & Peabody, 1987). Such approaches are more cost-effective than traditional extended hospitalizations and are suitable for many patients, but they require careful community development and adequate funding. Implementing comprehensive, compassionate, and cost-efficient health care delivery approaches for persons with AIDS will represent an ethical, political, and economic challenge for many years to come.

9.3. SPECIAL SENSITIVITIES REQUIRED OF AIDS CAREGIVERS

As implied in our discussion thus far, special therapist characteristics are needed in order to provide effective psychological and social care to persons affected by AIDS and HIV infection. Comfort when discussing sexuality and sexual behavior, nonjudgmental attitudes and ease when interacting with persons who are gay or have used intravenous drugs, and a willingness to consult comfortably with both traditional and nontraditional community organizations are essential. Continuing education programs can be used to disseminate accurate information on AIDS to "front-line" medical and social service professionals and to help alleviate apprehensions that might otherwise compromise the quality of care and relationships with patients (Kelly, St. Lawrence, Smith, Hood & Cook, 1987a; 1987b). Professionals are also likely to benefit from training programs that help them disentangle personal discomfort or disapproval from patient care responsibilities. While it would be naive to assume that all therapists can become equally comfortable in dealing with all patients, it is likely that many clinicians can be helped to become more comfortable and effective when working with AIDS-affected populations.

Professionals who care for AIDS patients face considerable stress in their work. At present, patients with full-blown AIDS invariably die, with the individual often suffering a recurrent and increasingly debilitating series of illnesses for which there are medical management regimens but no fundamental cures. It has been well established that most professionals in areas such as medicine, nursing, psychology, and social work are uncomfortable with dying persons and often avoid the terminally ill (Kübler-Ross, 1969). Caring for AIDS patients is even more psychologically draining for professionals because persons with AIDS are characteristically young, fear not only death but also debilitation and abandonment, and often face stresses in their relationships with family, friends, and others due to the stigma associated with AIDS. In many communities, clinics, and hospitals, professionals are either unwilling to see persons with AIDS or are uncomfortable doing so (Douglas & Calman, 1985; Searle, 1987). Consequently, those dedicated professionals who do see AIDS patents may find themselves overwhelmed (McKusick, Horstman, Abrams, & Coates, 1986). While the emotional drain is probably greatest for caregivers who see AIDS patients, professionals who work with persons exposed to HIV or those with HIV-related health problems other than frank AIDS have to accept the same uncertainties over the eventual health course of their clients that the clients themselves confront. The potential emotional toll in this area is great, both for the persons affected by HIV and for the sensitive professionals who care for them. Further, because AIDS itself elicits stigma, professionals who deal with AIDS patients or persons at risk may themselves be stigmatized, especially when they function in advocacy roles for persons affected by this disease.

It is exceedingly important that health care professionals who see persons with HIV illnesses develop support and coping methods for their own well-being, in much the same way that staff who treat other emotionally draining clients such as dying children or the terminally ill require stress-coping strategies. Professional peer support networks can assist AIDS-patient caregivers in better understanding and coping with feelings of frustration, helplessness, and depression. When caregivers who work with patients are themselves gay, fear and despair over seeing personal friends die of AIDS can be especially difficult. Strategies to minimize burnout, such as taking vacations, engaging in exercise, and allowing for leisure time, may need to be relearned and encouraged. It is important that workers in this area have available sources of counseling and other coping outlets to meet their own emotional needs. It is also useful for professionals who work frequently with end-stage AIDS patients to involve themselves in other activities, such as community prevention programs and services to persons who are HIV-positive but asymptomatic or with more mild symptoms. In this way, the therapist can direct attention to preserving health and promoting quality of life in addition to caring for those who are more seriously ill.

Epilogue
The Societal Challenge of AIDS

The primary focus of this book has been interventions that can prove useful in preventing AIDS and assisting persons already affected by the syndrome. The development of effective prevention and service delivery interventions—whether on an individual client, group, or community level—occupies the immediate attention of most therapists, social workers, and health care professionals who work in this area. However, beyond the care of current patients and beyond the development of behavior change strategies to prevent persons from becoming exposed to HIV infection, AIDS also presents challenges at a larger societal level to an extent that is unparalleled in modern times. The manner in which our political, judicial, educational, budgetary, research, and public health systems respond to the AIDS health crisis will determine the quality of health care that is available to persons with HIV illnesses, the quality of their lives, the success of education and prevention efforts, and the pace of biomedical research to prevent and cure HIV illnesses. As devastating as the health crisis has already been, every projection indicates that it will become much worse in all areas of the country and in all areas of the world.

It is by no means clear that our political, budgetary, and public health systems are geared to handle such large-scale emergencies. Early response to the AIDS health crisis by governmental, health, and research institutions has been characterized as slow, inadequate, and fragmented (Krieger & Appleman, 1986). Although AIDS research spending has increased substantially over the past several years, it still falls far short of the minimum funding levels recommended by national scientific panels and study groups (Committee on a National Strategy for AIDS of the Institute of Medicine, 1986). As discussed in Chapter 9, there are gaps in health care provision to persons with AIDS. Hospital and clinics in high prevalence areas are overwhelmed with patients who require intensive care but are often uninsured or minimally insured (Burda & Powills, 1986). AIDS patients in lower-prevalence areas, especially smaller cities, may find it impossible to obtain the medical and social support expertise they need. Some patients with AIDS die prematurely because they are unable to afford the costs of medications, such as AZT, which could extend their lives and reduce the need for even more expensive recurrent hospitalizations. Private, community, and "grass roots" volunteer organizations have often assumed the brunt of responsibility for developing needed services to AIDS patients. However, these community organizations are themselves becoming financially strapped and will certainly be unable to meet the needs of the rapidly growing population of AIDS-affected patients.

If one accepts the contention that research, prevention, political, and health care response to the AIDS crisis has been less vigorous and less adequate than what is needed, it behooves us to consider the reasons. There are a variety of possible explanations.

One explanation is that because most present AIDS patients are homosexual or bisexual males and intravenous drug users and because public attitudes toward homosexuals or drug users are generally negative, intolerant, and disdainful, many people may be unconcerned about their health (cf. Krieger & Appleman, 1986). There is unfortunately, empirical evidence suggesting that this is the case. AIDS patients are regarded by the public and even by some health care professionals as more deserving of their illnesses and as less deserving of medical care than patients with other serious diseases (Kelly, St. Lawrence, Smith, Hood, & Cook, 1987b; St. Lawrence et al., in press). AIDS patients who are homosexual are evaluated with greater negativity and prejudice than those who are heterosexual (St. Lawrence et al., in press). A recent study found that, in one geographical area, patients who acquired AIDS as a result of blood transfusions received 70% of the area's   total AIDS service budget, while patients who acquired AIDS through sexual contact or intravenous drug use were allocated only 30% in budgeted program funds, even though 90% of the patients fell into these latter groups (Flynn, Harper, *et al.*, 1987).

A related explanation for limited responsiveness to the health crisis involves the linkage of AIDS to sexual behavior. In the United States and in most European countries, religious, social, and cultural institutions stress the virtues of sexual abstinence until marriage and sexual fidelity following marriage. Because the development of AIDS is perceived to be a "consequence" of promiscuity, drug use, or other "vices," it becomes possible for some persons to view AIDS as an outcome—and even a deserved result—of patients' nonmonogamous sexual activity. Identified in the social psychological literature as "blaming the victim" (Temoshok, Sweet, & Zich, 1987), this perception can ultimately provide justifications for limiting care, utilizing the threat of AIDS to promote conservative social or religious agendas, or developing punitive responses toward persons who are viewed as culpable and deserving of their illnesses. While there have been no direct tests of how attitudes toward sexuality or how religious, or political, or moral conservatism influence attitudes concerning AIDS, advocacy groups for persons with the disease are convinced that such relationships exist (National Gay and Lesbian Task Force, 1987).

AIDS appeared in the United States at a time when deep cuts were being made in domestic spending programs. Reductions in the federal budgets available for biomedical and behavioral research, sex education, drug abuse prevention and treatment programs, public health, Medicaid, and health care services for the poor coincided with increased needs in all of these areas, owing to the emergence of AIDS. Unlike most other serious diseases with relatively stable prevalence rates, the number of persons affected by AIDS grows rapidly from year to year. Substantially increased AIDS research, treatment, and prevention expenditures now may avert an even greater economic catastrophe later. Funding for AIDS may also carry other benefits. Immunological and virological research on HIV infection could produce breakthroughs for the understanding and treatment of other serious diseases; changed sexual behavior produced by effective community-wide AIDS prevention programs could reduce the incidence of other sexually transmitted diseases and teenage pregnancies.

Efforts to combat AIDS have also been hindered by an inability to establish consensus concerning priorities and methods to best address the AIDS health crisis. Traditional methods of public health intervention for communicable diseases have been proposed and are being implemented in some areas. These traditional methods include making HIV infection a condition reportable to public health authorities, attempting to identify and track past sexual or needle-sharing partners of each HIV-seropositive individual, and then attempting to notify and track all of their past partners. While this model has been used with such easily treatable and rapid symptom-onset sexually transmitted diseases as syphilis and gonorrhea, it is unclear whether it will even prove feasible for persons with HIV infection who may be unable to identify all sexual partners over the past 10 years or more, who cannot currently be treated, and who may well remain infectious to sexual partners for their entire lives. In addition, fears of unsympathetic discrimination, ostracism, or even quarantine will limit the cooperation of many persons at risk for AIDS with public health programs they perceive as hostile, threatening, and unconcerned with their well-being.

An alternative public health approach—the development of wide-scale prevention and risk education programs focused on self-protection and targeted to children, adolescents, adults in the general population, and adult members of high-risk groups—has been proposed and advocated (U.S. Department of Public Health and Human Services, 1986a) but, for the most part, has not yet been implemented in the United States. To some degree, these delays appear to be the result of policy and philosophical disagreements concerning the content and scope of prevention messages. While virtually all authorities advocate abstinence, monogamy, and the avoidance of intravenous drugs as the only assured protections from HIV infection, it has been more difficult to reach a consensus on the explicitness needed in AIDS-prevention messages for those who are not monogamous, are not abstinent, or do use IV drugs. Because these are the groups at greatest risk for becoming exposed to HIV infection and for transmitting infection to others, they require the most aggressive, explicit, and prescriptive educational messages and prevention efforts. However, recommendations to counsel the sexually active in specific "safer sex" or risk-reduction guidelines, to teach current intravenous drug users how to sterilize needles, to prepare those adolescents who are sexually active to minimize their risk for AIDS, or even to advertise condoms meet with great resistance from those who argue that such steps advocate and condone promiscuity or drug use. As a result, prevention efforts urgently needed for populations at immediate risk often become paralyzed and greater numbers of people become HIV infected.

Finally, irrational fear and hysteria surround AIDS. There continue to be widespread fears that AIDS can be contracted during the course of everyday social contact with people who are HIV-infected, in spite of repeated studies that find no basis for such concerns. Children with asymptomatic HIV infection have been denied the right to attend school, and there are now widespread reports of unwarranted denial of employment, education, housing, transportation access, and health care to persons with AIDS or HIV infection. Although forceful action has occasionally been taken by some political, public health, and judicial leaders to counter public fears, correct misinformation, and prevent discrimination, many have chosen to remain silent.

It is, no doubt, easier to identify problems and barriers to effective responses to the AIDS health crisis than to implement solutions. Choices, however, will need to be made, and they will need to be made quickly if we are to avert a worldwide epidemic of perhaps unprecedented proportions. It is possible that societies will respond to the AIDS crisis with denial or with punitiveness, discrimination, hysteria, and scapegoating. Historically, these have been common societal responses to other health epidemics, and AIDS may trigger the same medieval responses (Mitchell, 1987). On the other hand, societies may choose to deal with this crisis differently by educating the public to reduce irrational fears about AIDS, by mobilizing scientific research resources in a focused and intensive manner, by implementing wide-scale prevention programs selected on the basis of their risk-behavior-change efficacy rather than their conformity to narrow social agendas, by protecting public health without abridging the rights of individuals, and by treating patients with compassion. Through our choices, we will make a statement that will be recorded and remembered across the ages.

Appendix
Selected AIDS Resources
in the United States

The organizations listed here are among those that conduct service programs for persons with AIDS, are involved in major AIDS-prevention campaigns, or serve as research and training resources. Most are able to provide materials related to AIDS at a nominal cost.

AID Atlanta
1132 W. Peachtree Street, N.W.
Atlanta, Georgia   30309
(404) 872-0600

AIDS Foundation of Houston
3927 Essex Lane
Houston, Texas   77027
(713) 623-6796

AIDS Project Los Angeles
3670 Wilshire Boulevard, Suite 300
Los Angeles, California   90010
(213) 738-8200

American College Health Association
15879 Crabbs Branch Way
Rockville, Maryland   20855
(301) 963-1100

American Foundation for AIDS Research
40 West 57th Street, Suite 406
New York, New York   10019-4001
(212) 556-9116

Gay Men's Health Crisis
P.O. Box 274
132 West 24th Street
New York, New York   10011
(212) 807-6655

Howard Brown Memorial Clinic
2676 N. Halsted
Chicago, Illinois   60657
(312) 975-0707

Mobilization Against AIDS
2120 Market Street, Suite 106
San Francisco, California   94114
(415) 431-4660

National AIDS Network
1012 14th Street, N.W., Suite 601
Washington, D.C.   20003
(202) 347-0390

National Association of People with AIDS
1012 14th Street, N.W., Suite 601
Washington, D.C.   20035
(202) 347-1317

National Gay Task Force
AIDS Information Line
1-800-221-7044

Public Health Service AIDS Hotline
1-800-342-2437

San Francisco AIDS Foundation
333 Valencia Street, 4th Floor
San Francisco, California   94103
(415) 863-2437

Shanti Project
890 Hayes Street
San Francisco, California 94114
(415) 558-9644

Whitman–Walker Clinic
1407 "S" Street N. W.
Washington, D.C. 20009
(202) 797-3500

References

Abdul-Quader, A. S., Friedman, S. R., Des Jarlais, D. C., Marmor, M., Maslansky, R., & Bartelme, S. (1987, June). *Behavior by intravenous drug users that can transmit HIV.* Paper presented to the III International Conference on AIDS, Washington, DC.

Abrams, D. I., Dilley, J. W., Maxey, L. M., & Volberding, P. A. (1986). Routine care and psychosocial support of the patient with the acquired immunodeficiency syndrome. *Medical Clinics of North America, 70,* 707–720.

Affleck, G., Tennen, H., Croog, S., & Levine, S. (1987). Casual attribution, perceived benefits, and morbidity after a heart attack: An 8-year study. *Journal of Consulting and Clinical Psychology, 55,* 29–35.

Alford, G. S. (1981). Hypnotics, sedatives, and minor tranquilizers. In S. J. Mulé (Ed.), *Behavior in excess: An examination of the volitional disorders.* New York: Macmillan Free Press.

Allen, S. R. (1984). Epidemiology of the acquired immunodeficiency syndrome (AIDS) in the United States. *Seminars in Oncology, 11,* 4–11.

Alter, M. J., Francis, D., & the CDC Sentinel County Study Group Centers for Disease Control. (1987, June). *Evidence of reduced AIDS associated risk behavior in homosexual/bisexual men but not in heterosexuals or IV drug users in 4 widely dispersed U.S. counties.* Paper presented to the III International Conference on AIDS, Washington, DC.

Anderson, R. E., & Levy, J. A. (1985). Prevalence of antibodies to AIDS-associated retrovirus in single men in San Francisco. *Lancet, 1,* 217.

Andrasik, F., Blanchard, E. B., Neff, D. F, & Rodichok, L. D. (1984). Biofeedback and relaxation training for chronic headache: A controlled comparison of booster treatments and regular contacts for long term maintenance. *Journal of Consulting and Clinical Psychology, 52,* 609–616.

Antoni, M. H. (1987). Neuroendocrine influences in psychoimmunology and neoplasis: A review. *Psychology and Health, 1,* 3–24.

Association of State and Territorial Health Officials Foundation. (1985). *Guide to public health practice: HTLV-III screening in the community.* Kensington, MD: Author.

Bandura, A. (1969). *Principles of behavior modification.* New York: Holt, Rinehart & Winston.

Bandura, A., & Walters, R. H. (1963). *Social learning and personality development.* New York: Holt, Rinehart & Winston.

Barnes, D. M. (1986). Grim projections for AIDS epidemic, *Science, 232,* 1589–1590.

Barre-Sinoussi, F., Chermann, S. C., Rey, Nugeyre, M. T., Chamaret, S., Gruest, J., Dauguet, C., Azler-Blin, C., Brun-Vezinet, F., Rouzioux, C., Rozenbaum, N., & Montagnier, L. (1983). Isolation of a T lymphotropic retrovirus from a patient at risk for acquired immune deficiency syndrome (AIDS). *Science, 220*(4599), 686–671.

Bartlett, E. E., Rabin, D., Taggart, V., Bandemer, C., & Bellonti, J. (1987, June). *Behavioral diagnosis for effective education of HIV-seropositive patients*. Paper presented to the III International Conference on AIDS, Washington, DC.

Bartnoff, H. S. (1987, June). *AIDS-HIV education for medical, nursing, and pharmacy students at the UCSF School of Medicine*. Paper presented to the III International Conference on AIDS, Washington, DC.

Bayer, H., Bienzle, U., Schneider, J., & Hunsmann, G. (1984). HTLV-III antibody frequency and severity of lymphadenopathy. *Lancet, 2*, 1347.

Bayer, R., Levine, C., & Murray, T. H. (1984). Guidelines for confidentiality in research on AIDS, *IRB, November/December* 1–7.

Bayer, R., Levine, C., & Wolf, S. M. (1986). HIV antibody screening: An ethical framework for evaluating proposed programs. *Journal of the American Medical Association, 256*(13), 1768–1774.

Bayer, R., Levine, C., & Wolf, S. M. (1987, June). *Confidentiality and the duty to protect: The limits of autonomy in the case of AIDS*. Paper presented to the III International Conference on AIDS, Washington, DC.

Bechtel, G. A. (1987, June). *Social support in gay men with the acquired immunodeficiency syndrome (AIDS)*. Paper presented to the III International Conference on AIDS, Washington, DC.

Beck, A. T. (1976). *Cognitive therapy and the emotional disorders*. New York: International Universities Press.

Beck, A. T., Rush, A. J., Shaw, B. F., & Emery, G. (1979). *Cognitive therapy of depression*. New York: Guilford Press.

Bickelhaupt, E. E. (1986). Psychosocial aspects of AIDS. *Kansas Medicine, March*, 66–68.

Billings, A. G., & Moos, R. H. (1982). Social support and functioning among community and clinical groups: A panel model. *Journal of Behavioral Medicine, 5*, 295–312.

Blattner, W. A., Biggar, R. J., Weiss, S. H., Melbye, M., & Goedert, J. J. (1985). Epidemiology of human T-lymphotropic virus type III and the risk of the acquired immunodeficiency syndrome. *Annals of Internal Medicine, 103*, 665–670.

Blattner, W. A., & Gallo, R. C. (1985). Human T-cell leukemia/lymphoma viruses: Clinical and epidemiologic features. *Current Topics in Microbiology and Immunology, 115*, 67–88.

Blattner, M., Goldberg, J., & Merbaum, M. (1978). Cognitive self-control factors in the reduction of smoking behavior. *Behavior Therapy, 9*, 553–561.

Bloom, J. R. (1982). Social support, accommodation to stress, and adjustment to breast cancer. *Social Science and Medicine, 16*, 1329–1338.

Boland, M., Keresztes, J., Evans, P., Oleske, J., & Connor, E. (1987, June). *HIV seroprevalence among nurses caring for children with AIDS/ARC*. Paper presented to the III International Conference on AIDS, Washington, DC.

Bovee, C. L., & Arens, W. F. (1986). *Contemporary advertising* (2nd ed.). Homewood, IL: Richard D. Irwin.

Boyko, W. J., Schecter, M. T., Jeffries, E., Douglas, B., Maynard, M., & O'Shaughnessy, M. (1985). The Vancouver lymphadenopathy-AIDS study: III. Relation of HTLV-III sero-positivity, immune status and lymphadenopathy. *Canadian Medical Association Journal, 133*, 28–32.

Brettle, R. P., Davidson, J., Davidson, S. J., Gray, J. M. N., Inglis, J. M., Conn, J. S., Bath, G. E., Gillon, J., & McClelland, D. B. L. (1986). HTLV-III antibodies in an Edinburgh clinic. *Lancet, 1*(8489), 1099.

Brigham, T. A. (1978). Cognitive self-control, part II. In A. C. Catania & T. A. Brigham (Eds.), *Handbook of applied behavior analysis: Social and instructional processes* (pp. 259–274). New York: Irvington.

Brondolo, E. N., Clemow, L. P., Saidi, P., & Lerner, A. (1987). *Psychosocial needs of hemophiliacs: A population at risk for AIDS*. Unpublished manuscript.

Browers, P., Hobak, M. C. Squillace, K., Joffe, R. T., & Rubinow, D. R. (1987, June). *Neuropsychological characterization of HIV infection*. Paper presented to the III International Conference on AIDS, Washington, DC.

Brown, G. R., Brandes, T., Haley, C., Seibert, G. B., Haley, R., & Anderson, R. (1987, June). *Costs of AIDS to a public hospital*. Paper presented to the III International Conference on AIDS, Washington, DC.

Brown, M. R. (1987). AIDS discrimination in the workplace: The legal dilemma. *Case and Comment, May–June*, 3–10.

Brownlee-Duffeck, L., Peterson, L., Simonds, J. F., Goldstein, D., Kilo, C., & Hoette, S. (1987). The role of health beliefs in the regimen adherence and metabolic control of adolescents and adults with diabetes mellitus. *Journal of Consulting and Clinical Psychology, 55*, 139–145.

Brundage, J. F., Burke, D. S., Gardner, L. I., Herbold, J., Voskovitch, J., & Redfield, R. R. (1987, June). *Temporal trend of prevalence and incidence of HIV infection among civilian applicants for US military service: Analysis of 18 months of serological screening data*. Paper presented to the III International Conference on AIDS, Washington, DC.

Brun-Vezinet, F., Rey, M. A., Katlama, C., Girad, P. M., Roulot, D., Yeni, P., Lemoble, L., Clavel, F., Alizon, M., Gradelle, S., Madjar, J. J., & Harzic, M. (1987). Lymphadenopathy-associated virus type II in AIDS and AIDS-related complex. *Lancet, 1*(8525), 128–132.

Buning, E. C. (1987, June). *Prevention policy on AIDS among drug addicts in Amsterdam*. Paper presented to the III International Conference on AIDS, Washington, DC.

Burda, D., & Powills, D. (1986). AIDS: A time bomb at hospitals' door. *Hospitals*, pp. 54–61.

Burish, T. G., Carey, M. P., Krozely, M. G., & Greco, F. A. (1987). Conditioned side effects induced by cancer chemotherapy: Prevention through behavioral treatment. *Journal of Consulting and Clinical Psychology, 55*, 42–48.

Calabrese, L. H., & Gopalakrishna, K. V. (1986). Transmission of HTLV-III infection from man to woman to man. *New England Journal of Medicine, 314*, 987.

Calabrese, L. H., Proffitt, M. R., Rehm, S., Lederman, M., Carey, J. T., Houser, H. B., Edmonds, K., & Ellner, J. J. (1985). Lack of correlation between promiscuity and seropositivity to HTLV-III from a low-incidence area for AIDS. *New England Journal of Medicine, 312*, 1256–1257.

Carlson, J. R., Bryant, M. L., Hinrichs, S. H., Yamamoto, J. K., Levy, N. B., Yee, J., Higgins, J., Levine, A. M., Holland, P., Gardner, M. B., & Pedersen, N. C. (1985). AIDS serology testing in low-and-high-risk groups. *Journal of the American Medical Association, 253*, 3405–3408.

Cass, V. S. (1979). Homosexual identity formation: A theoretical model. *Journal of Homosexuality, 4*, 219–235.

Castro, K. G., Lieb, S., Galisher, C., Witte, J., & Jaffe, H. W. (1987, June). *AIDS and HIV infection*. Paper presented to the III International Conference on AIDS, Washington, DC.

Cautela, J. R. (1966). A behavior therapy approach to pervasive anxiety. *Behaviour Research and Therapy, 4*, 99–111.

Cautela, J. R., & Bennett, A. K. (1981). Covert conditioning. In R. Corsini (Ed.), *Handbook of innovative psychotherapies*. New York: Wiley.

Cautela, J. R., & Wisocki, P. A. (1975). The thought stopping procedure: Description, application, and learning theory interpretations. *Psychological Record, 1*, 255–264.

Centers for Disease Control. (1981a). Pneumocystis pneumonia—Los Angeles. *Morbidity and Mortality Weekly Report, 30*, 250–252.

Centers for Disease Control. (1981b). Kaposi's sarcoma and pneumonia among homosexual men—New York City and California. *Morbidity and Mortality Weekly Report, 30*, 305–308.

Centers for Disease Control. (1983). Update: Acquired immunodeficiency syndrome (AIDS)—United States. *Morbidity and Mortality Weekly Report, 32*, 465–467.

Centers for Disease Control. (1985a). Current trends: Update on acquired immune deficiency syndrome (AIDS)—United States. *Morbidity and Mortality Weekly Report, 34,* 507–514.

Centers for Disease Control. (1985b). Summary: Recommendations for preventing transmission of infection with human T-lymphotropic virus type III/lymphadenopathy associated virus in the workplace. *Morbidity and Mortality Weekly Report, 35,* 334–339.

Centers for Disease Control. (1986a, November 17). *Acquired immunodeficiency syndrome (AIDS) weekly surveillance report: United States AIDS program.*

Centers for Disease Control. (1986b). Classification system for human T-lymphotropic virus type III/lymphadenopathy-associated virus infection—United States. *Morbidity and Mortality Weekly Report, 34,* 507–514.

Centers for Disease Control. (1986c). Human T-lymphotropic virus type III/lymphadenopathy-associated virus antibody testing at alternative sites. *Morbidity and Mortality Weekly Report, 35,* 284–287.

Centers for Disease Control. (1986d). Recommendations for preventing transmission of infection with human T-lymphotropic virus type III/lymphadenopathy-associated virus during invasive procedures. *Morbidity and Mortality Weekly Report, 35,* 221–223.

Centers for Disease Control. (1987, April 6). *Acquired immunodeficiency syndrome (AIDS) weekly surveillance: United States AIDS program.*

Chamberlain, M. E., Castro, K. G., Haverkos, H. W., Miller, B. I., Thomas, P. A., Reiss, R., Walker, J., Spira, T. J., Jaffe, H. W., & Curran, J. W. (1984). Acquired immunodeficiency syndrome in the United States: An analysis of cases outside high-incidence groups. *Annals of Internal Medicine, 101,* 617–623.

Chambless, D. D., & Goldstein, A. J. (1979). Behavioral psychotherapy. In R. J. Corsini (Ed.), *Current psychotherapies.* Itasca, IL: F. E. Peacock.

Ciobanu, N., & Wiernik, P. H. (1986). Malignant lymphomas, AIDS, and the pathogenic role of Epstein-Barr virus. *Mount Sinai Journal of Medicine, 53*(8), 627–633.

Clark, J. F., & McCallum, D. B. (1987, June). *The adequacy of hospital reimbursement for AIDS patients.* Paper presented to the III International Conference on AIDS, Washington, DC.

Clumeck, N., Sonnet, J., Taelman, H., Mascart-Lemone, F., DeBruyere, M., Van de Perre, P., Dashnoy, J., Marcelis, L., Lamy, M., Jonas, C., Eycksmans, L., Noel, H., Vanhaverbeek, M., & Butzler, J. P. (1984). Acquired immunodeficiency syndrome in African patients. *New England Journal of Medicine, 310,* 492–497.

Clumeck, N., Van de Perre, P., Carael, M., Rouvroy, D., & Nzaramba, D. (1985). Heterosexual promiscuity in African patients with AIDS. *New England Journal of Medicine, 313,* 182.

Coates, R. A., Calzavara, L., Read, S. E., Fanning, M. M., Shepherd, F. A., Klein, M. M., Johnson, J. K., & Soskolne, C. L. (1987, June). *Risk of HIV seropositivity in relation to specific sexual activities of sexual contacts of men with AIDS or ARC.* Paper presented to the III International Conference on AIDS, Washington, DC.

Coates, T. J., & McKusick, L. (1987, June). *The efficacy of stress management in reducing high risk behavior and improving immune function in HIV antibody positive men.* Paper presented to the III International Conference on AIDS, Washington, DC.

Coates, T. J., Morin, S. F., & McKusick, L. (1987, June). *Consequences of AIDS antibody testing among gay men: The AIDS behavioral research project.* Paper presented to the III International Conference on AIDS, Washington, DC.

Coates, T. J., Stall, R., Mandel, J. S., Boccellari, A., Sorensen, J. L., Morales, E. F., Morin, S. F., Wiley, J. A., & McKusick, L. (1987). AIDS: A psychosocial research agenda. *Annals of Behavioral Medicine, 9*(2), 21–28.

Coates, T. J., Temoshok, L., & Mandel, J. (1984). Psychosocial research is essential to understanding and treating AIDS. *American Psychologist, 39,* 1309–1314.

Cochran, S. D. (1987, June). *Psychosomatic distress and depressive symptoms among HTLV III/LAV seropositive, seronegative, and untreated homosexual men.* Paper presented to the III International Conference on AIDS, Washington, DC.

Cohen, M. A., & Weisman, H. W. (1986). A biopsychosocial approach to AIDS. *Psychosomatics, 27,* 245–249.

Cohen, S., & Willis, T. W. (1985). Stress, social support and the buffering hypothesis. *Psychological Bulletin, 98,* 310–357.

Colletta, N. D., Gregg, C. H., Hadler, S., Lee, D., & Mekelburg, D. (1980). When adolescent mothers return to school. *Journal of School Health, November,* 534–538.

Collier, A. C., Coombs, R. W., Nikora, B., Corey, L., & Handsfield, H. H. (1987, June). *Cerebrospinal fluid (CSF) findings in HIV-infected persons without clinically evident neurologic disease.* Paper presented to the III International Conference on AIDS, Washington, DC.

Collier, A. C. Murphy, V. L., Roberts, P. L., & Handsfield, H. H. (1987, June). *Clinical course of HIV seropositive homosexual men.* Paper presented to the III International Conference on AIDS, Washington, DC.

Committee on a National Strategy for AIDS of the Institute of Medicine. (1986). *Confronting AIDS: Directions for public health, health care, and research.* Washington, DC: National Academy Press.

Conant, M., Hardy, D., Sernatinger, J., Spicer, D., & Levy, J. A. (1986). Condoms prevent transmission of AIDS-associated retrovirus. *Journal of the American Medical Association,* 255(13), 1706.

Congressional Quarterly. (1987). Fighting AIDS: Congress looks for a way to help. February 14, pp. 263–267.

Cooke, M., & Koenig, B. (1987, June). *Housestaff attitudes toward the acquired immunodeficiency syndrome.* Paper presented to the III International Conference on AIDS, Washington, DC.

Cooper, D. A., Gold, J., MacLean, P., Donovan, B., Finlayson, R., Barnes, T. G., Michelmore, H. M., Brooke, P., & Penny, R. (1985). Acute AIDS retrovirus infection. Definition of a clinical illness associated with seroconversion. *Lancet,* 1(8428), 537–540.

Cousins, N. (1979). *Anatomy of an illness as perceived by the patient.* New York: Norton.

Crawford, L. (1987, June). *Comprehensive case management. Utilizing hospice concepts: A statement program.* Paper presented to the III International Conference on AIDS, Washington, DC.

Cupps, T. R., & Fauci, A. S. (1982). Corticosteroid-mediated immunoregulation in man. *Immunological Review, 65,* 133–150.

Curran, J. W. (1985). The epidemiology and prevention of acquired immunodeficiency syndrome. *Annals of Internal Medicine, 103,* 657–662.

Curran, J. W., Morgan, W. M., Starcher, E. T., Hardy, A. M., & Jaffe, H. W. (1985). Epidemiological trends of AIDS in the United States. *Cancer Research, 45,* 4602s–4604s.

Dax, E. M., Adler, W. H., Nagel, J. E., Dorsey, B. A., & Jaffe, J. H. (1987, June). *Amyl-nitrite inhalation alters immune function in normal volunteers.* Paper presented to the III International Conference on AIDS, Washington, DC.

Derogatis, L. R., Abeloff, M. D., & Melisaratos, N. (1979). Psychological coping mechanisms and survival time in metastatic breast cancer. *Journal of the American Medical Association,* 242, 1504, 1508.

Detels R., Fahey, J. L., Schwartz, K., Greene, R. S. Visscher, B. R., & Gottlieb, M. S. (1983). Relation between sexual practices and t-cell subsets in homosexually active men. *Lancet,* 1, 609–611.

Detels, R., Visscher, B., Kingsley, L., & Chmiel, J. (1987, June). *No HIV seroconversion among men refraining from anal–genital intercourse.* Paper presented to the III International Conference on AIDS, Washington, DC.

Devita, W. T., Hellman, S., & Rosenberg, S. A. (1985). *AIDS: Etiology, diagnosis, treatment, and prevention.* Philadelphia: J. B. Lippincott.

DiTullio, S. (1986). Editorial. *American Journal of Hospice Care, March/April,* 4.

Douglas, C. J., & Calman, C. M. (1985). Homophobia among physicians and nurses: An empirical study. *Hospitals and Community Psychiatry, 36,* 1309–1311.

Douglas, D. K., Harper, M., & Polk, F. (1987, June). *HIV positivity: The psychosocial impact of donor notification.* Paper presented to the III International Conference on AIDS, Washington, DC.

Drew, W. L. (1986). Is cytomegalovirus a cofactor in the pathogenesis of AIDS and Kaposi's sarcoma? *Mount Sinai Journal of Medicine, 53*(8), 622–625.

Drob, S., Bernard, H., Lifshutz, H., & Nierenberg, A. (1986). Brief group psychotherapy for herpes patients: A preliminary study. *Behavior Therapy, 17,* 2229–2238.

Drucker, E., McMaster, P., Wein, A., Bloom, J., Davis, R., & Alderman, M. B. (1987, June). *Hospital utilization patterns and charges for the care of inner city AIDS patients by risk group, sex, and race/ethnicity.* Paper presented to the III International Conference on AIDS, Washington, DC.

Drucker, E., & Vermund, S. H. (1987, June). *A method for estimating HIV seroprevalence rates in urban areas with high rates of I.V. drug abuse: The case of the Bronx.* Paper presented to III International Conference on AIDS, Washington, DC.

Dunkel-Schetter, C. (1984). Social support and adaptation to chronic illness: The case of maintenance hemodialysis. *Research in Nursing and Health, 2,* 101–108.

Dunkel-Schetter, C., & Wortman, C. B. (1982). The interpersonal dynamics of cancer: Problems in social relationships and their impact on the patient. In H. S. Friedman & M. R. DiMatteo (Eds.), *Interpersonal issues in health care* (pp. 349–381). New York: Academic Press.

Eales, L. J., Nyek, E., Parkin, J. M., Weber, J. N., Forest, S. M., Harris, J. R. W., & Pinching, A. J. (1987,May 2). Association of different allelic forms of group specific component with susceptibility to and clinical manifestation of human immunodeficiency virus infection. *Lancet,* 999–1002.

Ebbesen, P., Biggar, R. J., & Melbye, M. (1984). *AIDS: A basic guide for clinicians.* Copenhagen: Munksgaard.

Economist, The. (1987). American survey: No end to AIDS? *303* (June 6), 21–22.

Eisdorfer, C. (1987a, June). *Neuropsychiatric aspects of AIDS.* Paper presented to the III International Conference on AIDS, Washington, DC.

Eisdorfer, C. (1987b, June). *CNS complications of AIDS.* Paper presented to the III International Conference on AIDS, Washington, DC.

Ellis, A. (1984). *Rational-emotive therapy and cognitive-behavior therapy.* New York: Springer.

Ellis, A., & Grieger, R. (Eds.). (1977). *Handbook of rational emotive therapy.* New York: Springer.

Ellis, A., & Whiteley, J. M. (Eds.). (1979). *Theoretical and empirical foundations of rational emotive therapy.* Monterey, CA: Brooks/Cole.

Epstein, L. G., Share, L. R., Cho, E. S., Murphy-Cobb, M., & Baskin, G. B. (1987, June). *Comparative neuropathology of SIV and HIV brain infection.* Paper presented to the III International Conference on AIDS, Washington, DC.

Eskin, T. A., & Stoler, M. H. (1987, June). *Distribution of HIV message in postmortem brain.* Paper presented to the III International Conference on AIDS, Washington, DC.

Eyster, M. E., Goedert, J. J., Sarngadharan, M. G., Weiss, S. H., Gallo, R. C., & Blattner, W. A. (1985). Development and early natural history of HTLV-III antibodies in persons with hemophilia. *Journal of the American Medical Association, 253,* 2219–2223.

Fahrner, R., Clement, M. J., Kline, A., & Cohen, J. B. (1987, June). *Helping young people face death: Resuscitation status and outcome in first episode pneumocystis carinii pneumonia (PCP).* Paper presented to the III International Conference on AIDS, Washington, DC.

Fanning, M. M., Harmon, R., Shepherd, F. A., Vellend, H., & Minnick, S. (1987, June). *Influence of disease and case mix severity on the hospital costs of caring for AIDS patients.* Paper presented to the III International Conference on AIDS, Washington, DC.

Farthing, C. F., Jesson, W., Taylor, H-L., Lawrence, A. G., & Gazzard, B. G. (1987, June). *The HIV antibody test: Influence on sexual behavior of homosexual men.* Paper presented to the III International Conference on AIDS, Washington, DC.

Fauci, A. S. (1986). Current issues in developing a strategy for dealing with the acquired immunodeficiency syndrome. *Proceedings of the National Academy of Sciences, USA, 83,* 9278–9283.

Feinblum, S. (1986). Pinning down the psychosocial dimensions of AIDS. *Nursing and Health Care,* (7) 255–257.

Feldman, H. W., & Biernacki, P. (1987, June). *AIDS community outreach for intravenous drug users.* Paper presented to the III International Conference on AIDS, Washington, DC.

Feldman, I., Hummel, R. F., & Simmons, J. (1987, June). *Designated AIDS centers/AIDS intervention management systems (AIMS).* Paper presented to the III International Conference on AIDS, Washington, DC.

Felten, D. L., Felten, S. V., Carlson, S. L., Olschowka, J. A., & Livnat, S. (1985). Noradrenergic and peptidergic innervation of lymphoid tissue. *Journal of Immunology, 135,* 755–756.

Fischl, M. A., Dickinson, G. M., Scott, G. B., Klimas, N., Fletcher, M. A., & Parks, W. (1987). Evaluation of heterosexual partners, children, and household contact of adults with AIDS. *Journal of the American Medical Association, 257,* 640–644.

Fisher, E. J. (1986). How to combat the AIDS and FRAIDS epidemic. *Michigan Medicine, March,* 93–102.

Flynn, N. M., Harper, S., Jain, S., Holland, P., Fernando, L., & Bailey, V. (1987, June). *Underemphasis on publicly-funded programs for prevention of transmission of HIV among gay men and IV drug users.* Paper presented to the III International Conference on AIDS, Washington, DC.

Flynn, N. M., Jain, S., Harper, S., Bailey, B., Anderson, R., & Acuna, G. (1987, June). *Sharing of paraphernalia in intravenous drug users (IVDU): Knowledge of AIDS is incomplete and doesn't affect behavior.* Paper presented to the III International Conference on AIDS, Washington, DC.

Fox, P. C., & Baum, B. J. (1986). Isolation of HTLV-III virus from saliva in AIDS. *New England Journal of Medicine, 314,* 1307.

Fox, R., Ostrow, D., Valdiserri, R., Van Radden, M., Visscher, B., & Polk, B. F. (1987, June). *Changes in sexual activities among participants in the multicenter AIDS cohort study.* Paper presented to the III International Conference on AIDS, Washington, DC.

Francis, D. P., & Petriccian, J. C. (1985). The prospects for and pathways toward a vaccine for AIDS. *New England Journal of Medicine, 313,* 1586–1590.

Fredericksen, L. W., Solomon, L. G., & Brehony, K. A. (1984). *Marketing health behavior.* New York: Plenum.

Friedland, G. H., Kahl, P., Feiner, C., Rogers, M., Mayers, M., & Klein, R. S. (1987, June). *The effects of AIDS diagnosis upon close personal interactions among family members of AIDS patients.* Paper presented to the III International Conference on AIDS, Washington, DC.

Friedland, G. H., Saltzman, B., Rogers, M., Kahl, P., Feiner, C., & Mayers, M. (1987, June). *Additional evidence for lack of transmission for HIV infection to household contacts of AIDS patients.* Paper presented to the III International Conference on AIDS, Washington, DC.

Friedland, G. H., Saltzman, B. R., Rogers, M. F., Kahl, P. A., Lesser, M. L., Mayers, M. M., & Klein, R. S. (1986). Lack of transmission of HTLV-III/LAV infection to household contacts of patients with AIDS or AIDS-related complex with oral candidiasis. *New England Journal of Medicine, 314,* 344–349.

Funch, D. P., & Gale, E. N. (1984). Biofeedback and relaxation therapy for chronic temporomandibular joint pain: Predicting successful outcomes. *Journal of Consulting and Clinical Psychology, 52,* 928–935.

Funch, D. P., & Marshall, J. (1983). The role of stress, social support, and age in survival from breast cancer. *Journal of Psychosomatic Research, 27,* 77–83.

Funch, D. P., & Mettlin, C. (1982). The role of social support in relation to recovery from breast surgery. *Social Science and Medicine, 16,* 91–98.

Gadpaille, W. J. (1985). Homosexuality. In R. C. Simons (Ed.), *Understanding human behavior in health and illness* (pp. 391–401). Baltimore: Williams & Wilkins.

Gallo, R. (1987, June). *The AIDS viruses.* Paper presented to the III International Conference on AIDS, Washington, DC.

Gallo, R. C., Salahuddin, S. Z., Popovic, M., Shearer, G. M., Kaplan, M., Haynes, B. F., Palker, T. J., Redfield, R., Oleske, J., Safai, B., White, F., Foster, P., & Markham, P. D. (1984). Human T-lymphotropic retrovirus, HTLV-III, isolated from AIDS patients and donors at risk for AIDS. *Science, 224,* 500–503.

Garfield, C. (1978). *Psychosocial care of the dying patient.* New York: McGraw-Hill.

Gerald, G., Ramos, J., Bean, C., Rodriguez, G., Smith, W., & Sepulveda, J. (1987, June). *Communicating AIDS education across cultural barriers.* Paper presented to the III International Conference on AIDS, Washington, DC.

Gibbons, J., Parks, W., Parks, E., Hahn, B., & Shaw, G. (1987, June). *Genetic variations of the AIDS virus in vitro.* Paper presented to the III International Conference on AIDS, Washington, DC.

Godfried, J. P., Van Griensven, R. A. P., Tielamn, J., Goudsmit, J., Van der Noordaa, F., DeWolf, R. A., & Coutinho, R. A. (1987, June). *Effect of HIVab serodiagnosis on sexual behavior in homosexual men in the Netherlands.* Paper presented to the III International Conference on AIDS, Washington, DC.

Goedert, J. J. (1985). Recreational drugs: Relationship to AIDS. *Annals of the New York Academy of Sciences, 437,* 192–199.

Goedert, J. J., Biggar, R. J., Melbye, M., Mann, D. L., Wilson, S., Gail, M. H., Grossman, R. J., Digioia, R. A., Sanchez, W. C., Weiss, S. H., & Blattner, W. A. (1987). Effects of T4 count and cofactors on the incidence of AIDS in homosexual men infected with human immunodeficiency virus. *Journal of the American Medical Association, 257*(3), 331–334.

Goedert, J. J., & Blattner, W. A. (1985). The epidemiology of the acquired immunodeficiency syndrome. In V. T. Devita, S. Hellman, & S. A. Rosenberg, (Eds.), *AIDS: Etiology, diagnosis, treatment, and prevention* (pp. 1–30). Philadelphia: J. B. Lippincott.

Goedert, J. J., Sarngadharan, M. G., Biggar, R. J., Weiss, S. H., Winn, D. M., Grossman, R. J., Greene, M. H., Bodner, A. J., Mann, D. L., Strong, D. M., Gallo, R. C., & Blattner, W. A. (1984). Determinants of retrovirus (HTLV-III) antibody and immunodeficiency conditions in homosexual men. *Lancet, 2,* 711–716.

Goedert, J. J., Sarngadharan, M. G., Eyster, M. E., Weiss, S. H., Bodner, A. J., Gallo, R. C., & Blattner, W. A. (1985). Antibodies reactive with human T-cell leukemia viruses in the serum of hemophiliacs receiving factor VIII concentrate, *Blood, 65,* 492–495.

Gold, M., Seymour, N., & Sahl, J. (1986). Counseling HTLV-III seropositives. In L. McKusick (Ed.), *What to do about AIDS: Physicians and mental health professionals discuss the issues.* Berkeley: University of California Press.

Goldfried, M. R., & Davison, G. C. (1976). *Clinical behavior therapy.* New York: Holt, Rinehart & Winston.

Golubjatnikov, R., Pfister, J., & Tillotson, T. (1983). Homosexual promiscuity and the fear of AIDS. *Lancet, 1,* 681.

Gordon, L., & Zuckerman, C. (1987, June). *Multidisciplinary planning for the psychosocial and legal needs of persons with AIDS and their families.* Paper presented to the III International Conference on AIDS, Washington, DC.

Gottlieb, B. H. (1978). The development and application of a classification scheme of informal helping behaviors. *Canadian Journal of Science, 10,* 105–115.

Gottman, J., Notarious, C., Gonso, J., & Hartman, H. (1979). *A couple's guide to communication.* Champaign, IL: Research Press.

Grady, C., Jacob, J., Biard, B., Spross, J., & Ostchega, Y. (1987, June). *Identifying major concerns of patients with AIDS.* Paper presented to the III International Conference on AIDS, Washington, DC.

Green, J., Singer, M., & Wintfeld, N. (1987, June). *The AIDS epidemic: A projection of its impact on hospitals. 1986–1991.* Paper presented to the III International Conference on AIDS, Washington, DC.

Greer, S., Morris, T., & Pettingale, K. W. (1979). Psychological response to breast cancer: Effect on outcome. *Lancet, 2,* 785–787.

Gremminger, R. A. (1983). Taking a sexual history. *Wisconsin Medical Journal, 82,* 20–24.

Grimm, L. G. (1980). The evidence for cue-controlled relaxation. *Behavior Therapy, 11,* 282–293.

Groopman, J. E. (1985). Clinical spectrum of HTLV-III in humans. *Cancer Research, 45,* 4649s–4651s.

Groopman, J. E., Hartzband, P. I., Shulman, L., Salahuddin, S., Sarngadharan, M. G., McLane, M. F., Essex, M., & Gallo, R. (1985). Antibody seronegative human T-lymphotropic virus type III (HTLV-III)-infected patients with acquired immunodeficiency syndrome or related disorders. *Blood, 66* (3), 742–744.

Groopman, J. E., Mayer, K. H. , Sarngadharan, M. G., Ayotte, D., Devico, A. L., Finberg, R., Sliski, A. H., Allan, J. D., & Gallo, R. C. (1985). Seroepidemiology of human T-lymphotropic virus type III among homosexual men with the acquired immunodeficiency syndrome or generalized lymphadenopathy and among asymptomatic controls in Boston. *Annals of Internal Medicine, 102,* 334–337.

Groopman, J. E., Sarngadharan, M. B., Salahuddin, S. Z., Buxbaum, R., Huberman, M. S., Linniburgh, J., Sliski, A., Melane, M. F., Essex, M., & Gallo, R. C. (1985). Apparent transmission of human T-cell leukemia virus type III to a heterosexual woman with the acquired immunodeficiency syndrome. *Annals of Internal Medicine, 102,* 63–66.

Guinan, M. E., Thomas, P. A., Pinsky, P. F., Goodrich, J. T., Selik, R. M., Jaffe, H. W., Haverkos, H. W., Noble, G., & Curran, J. W. (1984). Heterosexual and homosexual patients with the acquired immunodeficiency syndrome. *Annals of Internal Medicine, 100,* 213–218.

Hackett, T. P., & Cassem, N. H. (1970). Psychological reactions to life-threatening illness. In H. Abrams, (Ed.), *Psychological aspects of stress.* Springfield, IL: Charles C Thomas.

Hackett, T. P., & Weisman, A. D. (1969). Denial as a social factor in patients with heart disease and cancer. *Annals of the New York Academy of Sciences, 164,* 802.

Halonen, J. S., & Passman, R. H. (1985). Relaxation and expectation in the treatment of postpartum distress. *Journal of Consulting and Clinical Psychology, 53,* 839–845.

Hammen, C. L., Jacobs, M., Mayol, A., & Cochran, D. S. (1980). Dysfunctional cognitions and the effectiveness of skills and cognitive-behavioral assertion training. *Journal of Consulting and Clinical Psychology, 48,* 685–695.

Harper, S., Flynn, N., Van Horne, J., Jain, S., Carlson, J., & Pollet, S. (1987, June). *Absence of HIV antibody among dental professionals, surgeons, and household contact exposed to persons with HIV infection.* Paper presented to the III International Conference on AIDS, Washington, DC.

Harris, C., Butkus-small, C. B., Klein, R. S., Friedman, E. H., Moll, B., Emerson, E. E., Spigland, I., & Steigbigel, N. H. (1983). Immunodeficiency in female sexual partners of men with the acquired immunodeficiency syndrome. *New England Journal of Medicine, 308,* 1181–1184.

Haverkos, H. W., & Drotman, D. P. (1984). The epidemiology of the acquired immunodeficiency syndrome. *Diagnostic Immunology, 2,* 67–72.

Hazaleus, S. L., & Deffenbacher, J. L. (1986). Relaxation and cognitive treatments of anger. *Journal of Consulting and Clinical Psychology, 54,* 222–226.

Herman, P. A. (1986). Neurologic effects of HTLV-III infection in adults: An overview. *Mount Sinai Journal of Medicine, 53*(8), 616–621.

Hersen, M., Eisler, R. M., Miller, P. M., Johnson, M. B., & Pinkston, S. G. (1973). Effects of practice, instructions, and modeling on components of assertive behavior. *Behaviour Research and Therapy, 11,* 443–451.

Hersen, M. Kazdin, A. E., Bellack, A. S., & Turner, S. M. (1979). Effects of live modeling, covert modeling, and rehearsal on assertiveness in psychiatric patients. *Behaviour Research and Therapy, 17,* 369–377.

Heseltine, P. N. R., Leedom, J. M., Hedderman, M., Ripper, M., & Sattler, F. (1987, June). *Comprehensive outpatient-based healthcare reduces inpatient stay for persons with AIDS or ARC: The Los Angeles County model.* Paper presented to the III International Conference on AIDS, Washington, DC.

Hessol, N. A., Rutherford, G. W., O'Malley, P. M., Doll, L. S., Darrow, W. W., & Jaffe, H. W. (1987, June). *The natural history of human immunodeficiency virus infection in a cohort of homosexual and bisexual men: A 7-year prospective study.* Paper presented to the III International Conference on AIDS, Washington, DC.

Hirsch, D. A., & Enlow, R. W. (1986). The effects of the acquired immune deficiency syndrome on gay lifestyle and the gay individual. *Annals of the New York Academy of Sciences, 437,* 273–282.

Ho, D. D., Byington, R. E., Schooley, R. T., Flynn, T., Rota, T. R., & Hirsh, M. S. (1985). Infrequency of isolation of HTLV-III virus from saliva in AIDS. *New England Journal of Medicine, 313,* 1606.

Ho, D. D., Rota, T. R., Schooley, R. T., Kaplan, J. C., Allan, J. D., Groopman, J. E., Resnick, L., Felsenstein, D., Andrews, C. A., & Hirsh, M. (1985). Isolation of HTLV-III from cerebrospinal fuid and neural tissue of patients with neurologic syndromes related to the acquired immunodeficiency syndrome. *New England Journal of Medicine, 313,* 1493–1497.

Hoelscher, T. J., Lichstein, K. L., Fischer, S., & Hegarty, T. B. (1987). Relaxation treatment of hypertension: Do home relaxation tapes enhance treatment outcome? *Behavior Therapy, 18,* 33–37.

Holland, J., & Tross, S. (1985). The psychosocial and neuropsychiatric sequelae of the acquired immunodeficiency syndrome and related disorders. *Annals of Internal Medicine, 103,* 760–764.

Hopkins, D. R. (1987a). Prevention of HIV Infection. *Journal of the American Medical Association, 257*(8), 1046.

Hopkins, D. R. (1987b, June). *Public health measures for prevention and control of AIDS.* Paper presented to the III International Conference on AIDS, Washington, DC.

Hospitals. (1986). DC insurers barred from testing for AIDS. July 5, pp. 50–51.

Hurzeler, R. J., & Rawson, D. (1987, June). *A hospice's response to the AIDS dilemma.* Paper presented to the III International Conference on AIDS, Washington, DC.

Jacobson, M. E. (1938). *Progressive relaxation.* Chicago: University of Chicago Press.

Jacobson, N. S., & Margolin, G. (1979). *Marital therapy: Strategies based on social learning and behavior exchange principles.* New York: Brunner/Mazel.

Jacobson, P. B., Perry, S. W., Scavuzzo, D., & Robert, R. B. (1987, June). *Psychological reactions of individuals at risk for AIDS during an experimental drug trial.* Paper presented to the III International Conference on AIDS, Washington, DC.

Jaffe, H. W., Bregman, D. J., & Selik, R. M. (1985). Acquired immune deficiency syndrome in the United States: The first 1000 cases. *Journal of Infectious Diseases, 148,* 339–345.

Jaffe, H. W., Choi, K., Thomas, P. A., Haverkos, J. W., Anerbach, D. M., Guinan, M. E., Rogers, M. F., Spira, T. J., Darrow, W. W., Kramer, M. A., Friedman, S. M., Monroe, J. M., Friedman-Kien, A. E., Laubenstein, L. J., Marmon, M., Safai, B., Dritz, S. K., Crisp, S. J., Fannin, S. L., Orkwis, J. F., Kelter, A., Rushing, W. R., Thacker, S. B., & Curran, J. W. (1983). National case-control study of Kaposi's sarcoma and pneumocystis carinii pneumonia in homosexual men: Part 1. Epidemiologic results. *Annals of Internal Medicine, 99,* 145–151.

Jaffe, H. W., Darrow, W. W., Echenberg, D. F., O'Malley, P. M., Getchell, J. P., Kalyanaram, V. S., Byers, R. H., Drennan, D. P., Braff, E. H., Curran, J. N., & Francis, D. P. (1985). The acquired immunodeficiency syndrome in a cohort of homosexual men. *Annals of Internal Medicine, 103,* 210–214.

Jaffe, H. W., Hardy, A. M., Morgan, W. M., & Darrow, W. W. (1985). The acquired immunodeficiency syndrome in gay men. *Annals of Internal Medicine, 103,* 662–664.

Jain, S., Flynn, N., Keddie, E., Carlson, J., Harper, S., & Bailey, V. (1987, June). *Disinfection of IV drug paraphernalia using commonly available materials: Hope for controlling spread of HIV among IV drug users?* Paper presented to the III International Conference on AIDS, Washgton, DC.

Janoff-Bulman, R., & Frieze, I. (1983). A theoretical perspective for understanding reactions to victimization. *Journal of Social Issues, 39,* 1–17.

Janssen, R. S., Saykin, A., Kaplan, J., Spira, T., Pinsky, P., & Schonberger, L. (1987, June). *Neurologic and neuropsychologic complications of lymphadenopathy syndrome.* Paper presented to the III International Conference on AIDS, Washington, DC.

Jay, S. M., Elliott, C., & Varni, J. W. (1986). Acute and chronic pain in adults and children with cancer. *Journal of Consulting and Clinical Psychology, 54*, 601–607.

Johnson, D., & McGrath, H. M. (1987, June). *Perceived changes in sexual practices among homosexual men.* Paper presented to the III International Conference on AIDS, Washington, DC.

Joseph, J. G., Montgomery, S., Kessler, R. C., Ostrow, D. G., Emmons, C. A., & Phair, J. P. (1987, June). *Two-year longitudinal study of behavioral risk reductions in a cohort of homosexual men.* Paper presented to the III International Conference on AIDS, Washington, DC.

Joseph, S. C. (1986). Justice Department opinion on AIDS: Another example of insensitivity (Editorial). *Hospital Practice*, September 15, p. 10.

Journal of the American Medical Association. (1985). Council on Scientific Affairs (1985) status report on the acquired immunodeficiency syndrome human T-cell lymphotropic virus type III testing, *254*, 1342–1345.

Journal of the American Medical Association. (1987a). Risk factors for AIDS among Haitians residing in the United States: Evidence of heterosexual transmission: The Collaborative Study Group of AIDS in Haitian-Americans, *257*, 635–639.

Journal of the American Medical Association. (1987b). Positive HTLV-III/LAV antibody results for sexually active female members of social/sexual clubs—Minnesota, *257*, 293–296.

Kaplan, H. B. (1980). Self esteem and self derogation theory of drug abuse. In *Theories on drug abuse: Selected contemporary perspectives.* NIDA Research Monograph. Washington, DC: U.S. Government Printing Office.

Kaplan, H. B., Robbins, C., & Martin, S. S. (1983). Antecedents of psychological stress in young adults: Self rejection, deprivation of social support, and life events. *Journal of Health and Social Behavior, 24*, 230–244.

Katchadourian, H. A., & Lunde, D. T. (1972). *Fundamentals of human sexuality.* New York: Holt, Rinehart & Winston.

Katlana, C., Rey, D., Salmon, P., Ngovan, P., & Dazza, M. C. (1987, June). *Cerebrospinal fluid (CSG) study in forty-five HIV infected patients: Clinical correlation with three isolation and intrathecal specific antibodies synthesis.* Paper presented to the III International Conference on AIDS, Washngton, DC.

Katz, A. H., & Bender, E. I. (1976). Self-help in society—The motif of mutual aid. In A. Katz & E. Bender (Eds.), *The strength in us: Self help groups in the modern world* (pp. 2–13). New York: New Viewpoints.

Katzenstein, D. A., Latif, A., Bassett, M. T., & Emmanuel, J. C. (1987, June). *Risks for heterosexual transmission of HIV in Zimbabwe.* Paper presented to the III International Conference on AIDS, Washington, DC.

Kaufman, N. J., Vergeront, J., & Frisby, H. (1987, June). *Ethical dilemmas inherent in HIV antibody testing legislation: A one year retrospective.* Paper presented to the III International Conference on AIDS, Washington, DC.

Kegels, S., Catania, J., & Coates, T. J. (1987, June). *Motivations and consequences of AIDS antibody testing among heterosexuals.* Paper presented to the III International Conference on AIDS, Washington, DC.

Kelly, J. A. (1982). *Social skills training: A practical guide for interventions.* New York: Springer.

Kelly, J. A. & St. Lawrence, J. S. (1986). Behavioral intervention and AIDS. *Behavior Therapist, 6*, 121–125.

Kelly, J. A., & St. Lawrence, J. S. (1987a). Cautions about condoms in prevention of AIDS. *Lancet, 1* (8528), 323.

Kelly, J. A., & St. Lawrence, J. S. (1987b). The prevention of AIDS: Roles for behavioral intervention. *Scandinavian Journal of Behaviour Therapy, 16*, 5–19.

Kelly, J. A., St. Lawrence, J. S., Brasfield, T. L., & Hood, H. V. (1987, June). *Relationships between knowledge about AIDS risk and actual risk behavior in a sample of homosexual men: Some implications for prevention.* Paper presented to the III International Conference on AIDS, Washington, DC.

Kelly, J. A., St. Lawrence, J. S., Hood, H. V., & Brasfield, T. L. (1987). *Behavioral intervention to reduce AIDS risk activities.* Manuscript submitted for review.

Kelly, J. A., St. Lawrence, J. S., Hood, H. V., Smith, S., Jr., & Cook, D. J. (in press). Nurses attitudes toward AIDS. *Journal of Continuing Education in Nursing.*

Kelly, J. A., St. Lawrence, J. S., Smith, S., Jr., Hood, H. V., & Cook, D. J. (1987a). Medical students' attitudes toward AIDS. *Journal of Medical Education, 62,* 549–556.

Kelly, J. A., St. Lawrence, J. S., Smith, S., Jr., Hood, H. V., & Cook, D. J. (1987b). Stigmatization of AIDS patients by physicians. *American Journal of Public Health, 77*(7), 789–791.

Kessler, R. C., & McLeod, J. D. (1985). Social support and mental health in community samples. In S. Cohen & L. Syme (Eds.), *Social support and health* (pp. 219–240). New York: Academic Press.

Kiecolt-Glaser, J. K., & Glaser, R. (1987). Psychosocial moderators of immune function. *Annals of Behavioral Medicine, 9*(2), 16–20.

Kingsley, L., Detels, R., Kaslow, R., Polk, B. F., Rinaldo, C. R., Jr., Chmiel, J., Detre, K., Kelsey, S. F., Odaka, K., Ostrow, D., VanRaden, M., & Visscher, B. (1987). Risk factors for seroconversion to human immunodeficiency virus among male homosexuals. *Lancet, 1*(8529), 345–349.

Kinsey, A. C., Pomeroy, W. B., & Martin, C. E. (1948). *Sexual behavior in the human male.* Philadelphia: W. B. Saunders.

Klein, S. J., & Fletcher, W. (1987, June). *The importance of supportive interventions for caregiving family/friends during the AIDS crisis.* Paper presented to the III International Conference on AIDS, Washington, DC.

Kleppner, O., Russell, T., & Verrill, G. (1983). *Advertising procedure* (8th ed.). Englewood Cliffs, NJ: Prentice-Hall.

Komada, C., & O'Donnell, M. (1987, June). *AIDS and the college campus: A model prevention program.* Paper presented to the III International Conference on AIDS, Washington, DC.

Koocher, G. P. (1986). Coping with a death from cancer. *Journal of Consulting and Clinical Psychology, 54,* 623–631.

Kotler, P. (1983). *Principles of marketing* (2nd ed.). Englewood Cliffs, NJ: Prentice-Hall.

Kovacs, J. A., & Masur, H. (1984). Treatment of opportunistic infections. In P. Ebbesen, R. S. Biggar, & M. Melbye (Eds.), *AIDS—A basic guide for clinicians* (pp. 84–98). Copenhagen: Munksgaard.

Krantz, D., & Deckel, A. (1983). Coping with coronary heart disease and stroke. In T. Burish & L. Bradley (Eds.), *Coping with chronic diseases: Research and applications* (pp. 85–111). New York: Academic Press.

Krieger, N., & Appleman, R. (1986). *The politics of AIDS.* Oakland, CA: Frontline Pamphlets.

Kübler-Ross, E. (1969). *On death and dying.* London: Macmillan Press.

Kutzen, H. S. (1986). A community approach to AIDS through hospice: Louisiana program promotes high quality of life. *American Journal of Hospice Care, March/April,* 17–23.

Lance, L. (1975). Human sexuality course socialization: An analysis of changes in sexual attitudes and sexual behavior. *Journal of Sex Education and Therapy, 2,* 8–14.

Landesman, S. H., & Viera, J. (1983). Acquired immune deficiency syndrome (AIDS). *Archives of Internal Medicine, 143,* 2307–2309.

Lang, W., Anderson, R. E., Perkins, H., Grant, R. M., Lyman, D., Winkelstein, W., Jr., Royce, R., & Levy, J. A. (1987). The San Francisco Men's Health Study: II. Clinical, immunologic, and serologic findings in men at risk for AIDS. *Journal of the American Medical Association, 257*(3), 326–330.

Lange, M., Klein, E. B., Inada, Y., McKinley, G., Ramey, W., & Grieco, H. M. H. (1987, June). *Epidemiologic observations and predictive factors for AIDS in a cohort of New York homosexuals: 5 year follow-up.* Paper presented to the III International Conference on AIDS, Washington, DC.

Laurence, J., Brun-Vezinet, F., Schutzer, S. E., Rouzioux, C., Klatzmann, D., Barre-Sinoussi, F., Chermann, J. C., & Montagnier, L. (1984). Lymphadenopathy-associated viral antibody in AIDS. Immune correlations and definition of a carrier state. *New England Journal of*

Medicine, 311, 1269–1273.

Lehman, D. R., Ellard, J. H., & Wortman, C. B. (1986). Social support for the bereaved: Recipients' and providers' perspectives on what is helpful. *Journal of Consulting and Clinical Psychology, 54,* 438–446.

Leiderman, I. Z., Flesher, A. R., Shriver, K., Schaefler, B. A., Adelsberg, B. R., & Tam, M. R. (1987, June). *Detection of HIV core antigen in the cerebrospinal fluid (CSF) in patients within the AIDS spectrum.* Paper presented to the III International Conference on AIDS, Washington, DC.

Leventhal, H., Safer, M. A., & Panagis, D. M. (1983). The impact of communication on the self-regulation of health benefits, decisions, and behavior. *Health Education Quarterly;, 10,* 3–31.

Levine, A. M., Parkash, S., Gill, P. S., Krailo, M., Rarick, M. U., Loureiro, C., & Rasheed, S. (1987, June). *Natural history of HIV infection in a cohort of homosexual men from Los Angeles.* Paper presented to the III International Conference on AIDS, Washington, DC.

Levy, R. M., Bredesen, D. E., & Rosenblum, M. L. (1985). Neurological manifestations of the acquired immunodeficiency syndrome (AIDS): Experience at UCSF and review of the literature. *Journal of Neurosurgery, 62,* 475–495.

Lichtman, R. R., & Taylor, S. E. (1986). Close relationshyips and the female cancer patient. In B. L. Anderson (Ed.), *Women with cancer: Psychological perspectives* (pp. 233–256). New York: Springer-Verlag.

Lieb, L., Mascola, L., Woodard, L., McAllister, D., Giles, M., & Fannin, S. (1987, June). *Prevalence of HIV antibodies among intravenous drug users in Los Angeles.* Paper presented to the III International Conference on AIDS, Washington, DC.

Link, R. N., Feingold, A. R., Charap, M. H., Freeman, K., & Shelov, S. (1987, June). *Concerns of medical and pediatric house officers about acquiring AIDS from their patients.* Paper presented to the III International Conference on AIDS, Washington, DC.

Lowenstein, R. J., & Sharfstein, S. S. (1983–1984). Neuropsychiatric aspects of acquired immune deficiency syndrome. *International Journal of Psychiatric Medicine, 13,* 255–260.

Luborsky, L., Mintz, J., Brightman, V. J., & Katcher, A. H. (1976). Herpes simplex and moods, a longitudinal study. *Journal of Psychosomatic Research, 20,* 543–548.

Lundy, J., Raaf, J. W., Deakins, S., Wanebo, J. H., Jacobs, D. A., Tsung-Doo, L., Jacobowitz, D., Spear, C., & Oettgan, H. F. (1975). The acute and chronic effects of alcohol and the human immune system. *Surgery, Gynecology, and Obstetrics, 141,* 212–218.

Lyles, J. N., Burish, T. G., Krozely, M. G., & Oldham, R. K. (1982). Efficacy of relaxation training and guided imagery in reducing the adverseness of cancer chemotherapy. *Journal of Consulting and Clinical Psychology, 50,* 509–529.

Lyman, D., Ascher, M., & Levy, J. A. (1986). Minimal risk of transmission of AIDS-associated retrovirus infection by oral-genital contact. *Journal of the American Medical Association, 255,* 1703.

Lyons, C., Cossaboom, M., Graham, V., Honey, E., & Landesman, S. (1987, June). *The unique counseling intervention required for intravenous drug abusers (IVDAs) and their families.* Paper presented to the III International Conference on AIDS, Washington, DC.

Lyter, D. A., Valdiserri, L. A., Kingsley, W. P., Amoroso, C. R., & Rinaldo, J. R. (1987, June). *Factors influencing the decision to learn HIV antibody status in gay and bisexual men.* Paper presented to the III International Conference on AIDS, Washington, DC.

Maburn, G. T. (1982). Smoking: Introduction and overview. In T. J. Coates, A. C. Petersen, & C. Perry (Edss.), *Promoting adolescent health: A dialog on research and practice.* New York: Academic Press.

Macher, A. M., & Reichert, C. M. 91984). The pathological findings associated with opportunistic infections in AIDS. In P. Ebbesen, R. S. Biggar, & M. Melbye (Eds.), *AIDS—A basic guide for clinicians* (pp. 113–122). Copenhagen: Munksgaard.

Maisiak, R., Cain, M., Yarbro, C., & Josof, L. (1981). Evaluation of TOUCH: An oncology self-help group. *Oncology Nursing Forum, 8,* 10–25.

Mandel, J. S. (1985). *Affective reactions to a diagnosis of AIDS or ARC in gay men.* Unpublished doctoral dissertation, Wright Institute, Los Angeles.

Mandel, J. S., Coates, T. J., Wiley, J., Bart, T., & Woods, W. J. (1987, June). *Disclosure of health concerns and homosexuality among 671 men at risk of AIDS.* Paper presented to the III International Conference on AIDS, Washington, DC.

Mandel, J. S., Grade, M., Zegans, L. S., Bartnof, H., Faltz, B., & Ziegler, J. L. (1987, June). *A model for AIDS professional education.* Paper presented to the III International Conference on AIDS, Washington, DC.

Mandel, J. S., & Namir, S. (1986). Overview of treatment issues. In L. McKusick (Ed.), *What to do about AIDS: Physicians and mental health professionals discuss the issues* (pp. 78–91). Berkeley, CA: University of California Press.

Marcus, R., & the Cooperative Needlestick Surveillance Group. (1987, June). *Update: Prospective evaluation of health-care workers parenterally exposed to blood of patients infected with human immunodeficiency virus.* Paper presented to the III International Conference on AIDS, Washington, DC.

Marlink, R. G., Foss, B., Swift, R., Davis, W., Essex, M., & Groopman, J. (1987, June). *High rate of HTLV-III/HIV exposure in IVDA's from a small-sized city and the failure of specialized methadone maintenance to prevent further drug use.* Paper presented to the III International Conference on AIDS, Washington, DC.

Marmor, M. Friedman-Kien, A. E., Laubenstein, L., Byrum, R. D., William, D. C., D'Onofrio, S., & Dubin, N. (1982). Risk factors for Kaposi's sarcoma in homosexual men. *Lancet, 1,* 1083–1086.

Martin, J. P. (1986). The AIDS home care and hospice program: A multidisciplinary approach to caring for persons with AIDS. *American Journal of Hospice Care, March/April,* 35–37.

Martin, J. P. (1987, June). *Coming home hospice: A model residential hospice alternative.* Paper presented to the III International Conference on AIDS, Washington, DC.

Martinson, I. M., Nesbit, M., & Kersey, M. (1984). Home care for the child with cancer. In A. E. Christ & A. K. Flomenhaft (Eds.), *Childhood cancer: Impact on the family* (pp. 77–186). New York: Plenum.

Mathur-Wagh, U., Enlow, R., Spigland, I., Winchester, R. J., Sacks, H. S., Rorat, E., Yancovitz, S. R., Klein, M. J., William, D. C., & Mildvan, D. (1984). Longitudinal study of persistent generalized lymphadenopathy in homosexual men: Relation to acquired immunodeficiency syndrome. *Lancet, 1,* 1033.

Matthews, G. W., & Neslund, V. S. (1987). The initial impact of AIDS on public health law in the United States. *Journal of the American Medical Association, 257,* 344–352.

Mayer, K. H., Stoddard, A. M., McCusker, J., Ayotte, D., Ferriani, B. A., & Groopman, J. E. (1986). Human T–lymphotropic virus type III in high–risk, antibody negative homosexual men. *Annals of Internal Medicine, 104,* 194–196.

McAlister, A. (1984). Community studies of smoking cessation and prevention. In U. S. Department of Health and Human Services, *Health consequences of smoking for chronic obstructive lung disease: A report of the surgeon general.* Washington, DC: U.S. Government Printing Office.

McArthur, J. C., Farzadegan, H., Cornblath, D. R., Griffin, D.E., Johnson, R. T., & Folk B. F. (1987, June). *Cerebrospinal fluid abnormalities in homosexual/bisexual men with and without neuropsychiatric symptoms.* Paper presented to the III International Conference on AIDS, Washington, D. C.

McKusick, L., Horstman, W., Abrams, D., & Coates, T. J. (1986). The psychological impact of AIDS on primary care physicians. *Western Journal of Medicine, 144,* 751–752.

McKusick, L., Horstman, W., & Coates, T. J. (1985). AIDS and sexual behavior reported by gay men in San Francisco. *American Journal of Public Health, 75*(15), 493–496.

Meichenbaum, D. (1975). A self–instructional approach to stress management: A proposal for stress inoculation training. In C. Spielberger & J. Sarason (Eds.), *Stress and anxiety* (Vol. 2). New York: Wiley.

Meichenbaum, D. (1977). *Cognitive–behavior modification: An integrative approach.* New York: Plenum.

Meichenbaum, O., & Cameron, R. (1974). The clinical potential of modifying what clients say to themselves. *Psychotherapy: Theory, Research, and Practice, 11*, 103–117.

Meichenbaum, D., & Jaremko, M. E. (Eds.). (1983). *Steess reduction and prevention.* New York: Plenum.

Melbye, M., Biggar, R. J., Ebbesen, P., Sarngadharan, M. G., Weiss, S. H., Gallo, R. C., & Blattner, W. A. (1984). Seroepidemiology of HTLV-III antibody in Danish homosexual men: Prevalence, transmission, and disease outcome. *British Medical Journal, 289*, 573–575.

Merritt, R., Rowe, M., & Ryan, C. (1987, June). *AIDS: A public health challenge for states.* Paper presented to the III International Conference on AIDS, Washington, DC.

Miller, D., Jeffries, O. J., Green, J., Harris, J. R. W., & Pinching, A. J. (1986), HTLV-III: Should testing be routine? *British Medical Journal, 292*, 941–943.

Miller, P. M., & Foy, D. W. (1981). Substance abuse. In S. M. Turner, K. S. Calhoun, & H. E. Adams (Eds.), *Handbook of clinical behavior therapy* (pp. 191–213). New York: Wiley.

Mills, M., Wofsy, C. B., & Mills, J. (1986). The acquired immunodeficiency syndrome: Infection control and public health law. *New England Journal of Medicine, 314*, 931–936.

Mitchell, C., & Stuart, R. B. (1984). Effect of self-efficacy on dropout from obesity treatment. *Journal of Consulting and Clinical Psychology, 52*, 1100–1101.

Mitchell, D. J. (1987). *AIDS in historical perspective.* Unpublished manuscript, Jackson State University, Jackson, MS.

Mitsuya, H., Weinhold, K. J., Furman, A., St. Clair, M. H., Lehrman, S. N., Gallo, R. C., Bologwes, D., Barry, D. W., & Broder, S. (1985). 3'azido-3'deoxythymidine (BWA5096): An anti-viral agent that inhibits the infectivity and cytopathic effect of human T-lymphotropic virus type III/lymphadenopathy-associated virus in vitro. *Proceedings of the National Academy of Sciences, USA, 2*, 7096–7100.

Montagnier, L., Gruest, J., Chamaret, S., Dauguet, C., Axler, C., Guetard, D., Nugeyre, M. T., Barre-Sinoussi, F., Chermann, J. C., Brunet, J. B., Klatzmann, D., & Gluckmann, J. C. (1984). Adaptation of lymphadenopathy associated virus (LAV) to replication in EBV-transformed B-lymphoblastoid cell lines. *Science, 225*, 63–66.

Morin, S., Charles, K., & Malyon, A. K. (1984). Psychosocial impact of AIDS on gay men. *American Psychologist, 39*, 1288–1293.

Morin, S., Coates, T. J., Woods, W., & McKusick, L. (1987, June). *AIDS antibody testing: Who takes the test?* Paper presented to the III International Conference on AIDS, Washington, DC.

Morrow, G. R. (1984). Appropriateness of taped versus live relaxation in the systematic desensitization of anticipatory nausea and vomiting in cancer patients. *Journal of Consulting and Clinical Psychology, 52*, 1098–1099.

Moss, A. R., Osmond, D., Bacchetti, P., Casavant, C., Chermann, J. C., & Carlsen, J. (1987, June). *Three-year progression to clinical AIDS in seropositive men: The San Francisco General Hospital study.* Paper presented to the III International Conference on AIDS, Washington, DC.

Moulton, J. M., Sweet, D. M., Temoshok, L., & Mandel, J. S. (1987). Attribution of blame and responsibility in relation to distress and health behavior change in people with AIDS and AIDS-related complex. *Journal of Applied Social Psychology, 17*(5), 493–502.

Moynihan, R. T., McFarlane, R., Christ, G. H., Samet, R., Beckham, D., & Richardson, S. (1987, June). *An AIDS training program for mental health professionals.* Paper presented to the III International Conference on AIDS, Washington, DC.

Murphy, Sister P. (1986). Pastoral care and persons with AIDS. *American Journal of Hospice Care, March/April*, 38–40.

Myers, P. S. (1987). The impact of AIDS: A survey of large life and health insurers. *Journal of American Society of CLU and CHFC, May*, 72–78.

National Gay and Lesbian Task Force. (1987). *Anti-gay violence: Victimization and defamation in*

1986. New York: National Gay and Lesbian Task Force.

Nature. (1987). Who pays for AIDS?, *321,* 548.

Navia, B., & Price, R. (1986). Dementia complicating AIDS. *Psychiatric Annals, 19,* 82–85.

Neff, D. F., & Blanchard, E. B. (1987). A multi-component treatment for irritable bowel syndrome. *Behavior Therapy, 18,* 70–83.

Newell, G. R., Mansell, P. W., Wilson, M. B., Lynch, H. K., Spitz, M. R., & Hersh, E. M. (1985). Risk factor analysis among men referred for possible acquired immune deficiency syndrome. *Preventive Medicine, 14,* 81–91.

Newsweek. (1985). AIDS: A growing threat. August 12, pp. 40–47.

Nyanjom, D., Greaves, W., Delapenha, R., Barnes, S., Boynes, F., & Frederick W. R. (1987, June). *Sexual behavior change among HIV seropositive individuals.* Paper presented to the III International Conference on AIDS, Washington, DC.

Ockene, J. K., & Camic, P. M. (1985). Public health approaches to cigarette smoking cessation. *Annals of Behavioral Medicine, 7,* 14–18.

Oldenburg, B., Perkins, R. J., & Andrews, G. (1985). Controlled trial of psychological intervention in myocardial infarction. *Journal of Consulting and Clinical Psychology, 53,* 850–859.

Oleske, J., Minnefor, A., Cooper, R., Jr., Thomas, K., dela Cruz, A., Ahdieh, H., Guerrero, I., Joshi, V. V., & Desposito, F. (1983). Immune deficiency syndrome in children. *Journal of the American Medical Association, 249,* 2345–2349.

Orne, M. T., & Wender, P. H. (1968). Anticipatory socialization for psychotherapy: Method and rationale. *American Journal of Psychiatry, 124,* 1202–1212.

Osterweiss, M., Solomon, F., & Green, M. (Eds.). (1984). *Bereavement: Reactions, consequences, and care.* Washington, DC: National Academy Press.

Ottenberg, P. (1986). Public attitudes toward the control of AIDS: The homosexuals plight. *Transactions and Studies of the College of Physicians of Philadelphia, 8*(2), 113–122.

Padian, N., Wiley, J., & Winkelstein, W. (1987, June). *Male-to-female transmission of human immunodeficiency virus (HIV): Current results, infectivity rates, and San Francisco population seroprevalence estimates.* Paper presented to the III International Conference on AIDS, Washington, DC.

Parkes, C. M., & Weiss, R. (1983). *Recovery from bereavement.* New York: Springer-Verlag.

Penzien, D. B. (1986). The acquired immunodeficiency syndrome (AIDS): Essential information for mental health practitioners. *Behavior Therapist, 6,* 117–120.

Perry, J., Rogriguez, G., Rotkiewicz, L., & Young, S. (1987, June). *A conceptual model for a transitional self-help residence of IVDA with AIDS/ARC.* Paper presented to the III International Conference on AIDS, Washington, DC.

Perry, S. W., & Tross, S. (1984). Psychiatric problems of AIDS inpatients at the New York Hospital: Preliminary report. *Public Health Reports, 99,* 200–205.

Peterman, T. A., Jaffe, H. W., Feorino, P. M., Getchell, J. P., Warfield, D. T., Haverkos, H. W., Stoneburner, R. L., & Curran, J. W. (1985). Transfusion-associated acquired immunodeficiency syndrome in the United States. *Journal of the American Medical Association, 254,* 2913–2917.

Pickles, H., & Bond, G. (1987, June). *Assessment of the AIDS public information campaign in the UK.* Paper presented to the III International Conference on AIDS, Washington, DC.

Piot, P., Quinn, T. C., Taelman, H., Feinsod, F. M., Minlangu, K. B., Wobin, O., Mbendi, N., Mazebo, P., Ndangi, K., Stevens, W., Kalambayi, K., Mitchell, S., Bridts, C., & McCormick, J. B. (1984). Acquired immunodeficiency syndrome in a heterosexual population in Zaire. *Lancet, 2,* 65–69.

Plotkin-Israel, I. (1984). *Causal attributions, perceived control, and coping among MI patients.* Paper presented at the annual meeting of the American Psychological Association, Toronto, Canada.

Plummer, F. A., Simonsen, J. N., Ngugi, E. N., Cameron, D. W., Piot, P., Ndinya-Achola, J. (1987, June). *Incidence of human immunodeficiency virus (HIV) infection and related disease in a cohort of Nairobi prostitutes.* Paper presented to the III International Conference on AIDS, Washington, DC.

Polis, M. A., Polk, B. F., Phair, J. P., Rinaldo, C. R., Nishanian, P., & Saab, A. J. (1987, June). *Reversion of HIV serology from positive to negative in gay/bisexual men who remain healthy.* Paper presented to the III International Conference on AIDS, Washington, DC.

Polk, B. F., Fox, R., Brookmeyer, R., Kanchanaraksa, S., Kaslow, R., Visscher, B., Rinaldo, C., & Phair, J. P. (1987). Predictors of the acquired immunodeficiency syndrome developing in a cohort of seropositive homosexual men. *New England Journal of Medicine, 316,* 61–66.

Pollak, M., Gharakhanian, C., Rozenbaum, W., Viallefont, A., & Aine, F. (1987, June). *An unspeakable disease: Self isolation of HIV infected patients as a result of conflicting aspirations.* Paper presented to the III International Conference on AIDS, Washington, DC.

Pomeroy, W. B., Flax, C. C., & Wheeler, C. C. (1982). *Taking a sex history.* New York: Free Press.

Quadland, M., Shattls, W. D., Schuman, R., & Jacobs, R. (1987, June). *The 800 men study: A controlled study of an AIDS prevention program in New York City.* Paper presented to the III International Conference on AIDS, Washington, DC.

Rando, R. A. (1983). An investigation of grief and adaptation in parents whose children have died from cancer. *Journal of Pediatric Psychology, 8,* 3–20.

Redfield, R. R., Markham, P. D., Salahuddin, S. Z., Wright, D. C., Sarngadharan, M. G., & Gallo, R. C. (1987). Heterosexually acquired HTLV-III/LAV disease (AIDS-related complex and AIDS): Epidemiologic evidence for female-to-male transmission. *Journal of the American Medical Association, 254,* 2094–2096.

Reed, P., Wise, T. N., & Mann, L. S. (1984). Nurses' attitudes regarding acquired immunodeficiency syndrome (AIDS). *Nursing Forum, 4,* 153–156.

Rietmeijer, C., Krebs, J. W., Feorino, P. M., & Judson, F. N. (1987, June). *In vitro tests demonstrate condoms containing nonoxynol-9 provide effective physical and chemical barriers against human immunodeficiency virus.* Paper presented to the III International Conference on AIDS, Washington, DC.

Robert-Guroff, M., Weiss, S. H., Giron, J. A., Jennings, A. M., Ginzburg, H. M., Margolis, I. B., Blattner, W. A., & Gallo, R. E. (1986). Prevalence of antibodies to HTLV-I, -II and -III in intravenous drug abusers from an AIDS endemic region. *Journal of the American Medical Association, 255,* 3133–3137.

Rodriguez, G., & Jackson, J. (1987, June). *AIDS medical day care for intravenous drug abusers.* Paper presented to the III International Conference on AIDS, Washington, DC.

Rogentine, G. N., Fox, B. H., VanKammen, D. P., Rosenblatt, J., Docherty, J. P., & Bunney, W. E. (1979). Psychological and biological factors in the short term prognosis of malignant melanoma. *Psychiatric Medicine, 41,* 647–655.

Rosen, J. C., & Solomon, L. J. (1985). *Prevention in health psychology.* Hanover, NH: University Press of New England.

Rosenburg, M. (1965). *Society and the adolescent self-image.* Princeton, NJ: Princeton University Press.

Rubenstein, A., Sicklick, M., Gupta, A., Berstein, L., Klein, N., Rubinstein, E., Spigland, I., Fruchter, L., Litman, N., Lee, H., & Hollander, M. (1983). Acquired immunodeficiency with reversed T4/T8 ratios in infants born to promiscuous and drug-addicted mothers. *Journal of the American Medical Association, 249,* 2350–2356.

Ruff, M. R., Hill, J., Smith, C., Hallberg, P., Sternberg, E., Jelesoff, N., O'Neill, J. B., & Pert, C. B. (1987, June). *Neuropeptides and the HIV receptor: Peptide T 4–8 and its pentapeptide analogues are potent CO4 receptorligands present in sera of all HIV isolates.* Paper presented to the III International Conference on AIDS, Washington, DC.

Sackett, D. L., Haynes, R. B., Gibson, E. S., Hackett, B. C., Taylor, D. W., Roberts, R. S., & Johnson, A. C. (1975). Randomized clinical trial of strategies for improving medication compliance in primary hypertension. *Lancet, 1,* 1205–1207.

Safai, B., Sarngadharan, M. G., Groopman, J. E., Arnett, K., Popovic, M., Sliski, A., Schupbach,

J., & Gallo, R. C. (1984). Seroepidemiological studies of human T-lymphotropic retrovirus type III in acquired immunodeficiency syndrome. *Lancet, 1,* 1438–1440.

Scesney, S. M., Gantz, N. M., & Sullivan, J. L. (1987, June). *Impermeability of condoms to HIV and inactivation of HIV by the spermacide nonocynol-9.* Paper presented to the III International Conference on AIDS, Washington, DC.

Schatz, B. (1987, June). *Legal and ethical analysis of insurance underwriting for AIDS.* Paper presented to the III International Conference on AIDS, Washington, DC.

Schechter, M. T., Boyko, W. J., Weaver, M. S., Douglas, B., Willoughby, B., & McLeod, W. A. (1987, June). *Progression to AIDS, predictors of AIDS, and seroconversion in a cohort of homosexual men: Results of a four year prospective study.* Paper presented to the III International Conference on AIDS, Washington, DC.

Schechter, M. T., Jeffries, E., Constance, P., Douglas, B., Fay, S., Maynard, M., Nitt, R., Willoughby, B., Boyko, W. J., & McLeod, W. A.(1984). Changes in sexual behavior and fear of AIDS. *Lancet, 1,* 1293.

Schietinger, H., Fitzhugh, Z. A., McCarthy, P. K., & Morrison, C. (1987, June). *AIDS train the trainer program for health care providers: California Nurses Association's innovative approach.* Paper presented to the III International Conference on AIDS, Washington, DC.

Schofferman, J. (1986). Medicine and the psychology of treating the terminally ill. In L. McKusick (Ed.), *AIDS and mental health: Policy, administration, treatment.* San Francisco: AIDS Clinical Research Center.

Schorr, J. B., Berkowitz, A., Cumming, P. D., Katz, A. J., & Sandler, S. G. (1985). Prevalence of HTLV-III antibody in American blood donors. *New England Journal of Medicine, 313,* 384–385.

Schulman, D. I., Karp, M., & Nickens, N. (1987, June). *Municipal AIDS discrimination laws as public health education tools for preventing HIV transmission.* Paper presented to the III International Conference on AIDS, Washgton, DC.

Seage, G. R., Landers, S., Barry, A., Lamb, G., & Epstein, A. (1987, June). *Cost of medical care for AIDS in Massachusetts: Trends over a two year period.* Paper presented to the III International Conference on AIDS, Washington, DC.

Seale, J. (1985). AIDS virus infection: Prognosis and transmission. *Journal of the Royal Society of Medicine, 78,* 613–615.

Searle, E. S. (1987). Knowledge, attitudes, and behavior of health professionals in relation to AIDS. *Lancet, 1,* 26–28.

Seidel, L., & Goebel, F. (1987, June). *Psychological problems in nursing patients with AIDS.* Paper presented to the III International Conference on AIDS, Washington, DC.

Selik, R. M., & Rogers, M. F. (1987, June). *Relative risk of AIDS for American blacks and Hispanics.* Paper presented to the III International Conference on AIDS, Washington, DC.

Selye, H. (1946). The general application syndrome and the diseases of adaptation. *Journal of Clinical Endocrinology, 6,* 117.

Selye, H. (1956). *The stress of life.* New York: McGraw-Hill.

Sidtis, J. J., Amitai, H., Ornitz, D., & Price, R. W. (1987, June). *The brief neuropsychological examination for AIDS dementia complex: Correlations with functional status scales and other neuropsychological tests.* Paper presented to the III International Conference on AIDS, Washington, DC.

Siegal, F. P., Lopez, C., Fitzgerald-Bocarsly, P. A., Zito, J. L., Reife, R., & Cheung, T. W. (1987, June). *Immunologic status of patients with chronic progressive HIV encephalomyelopathy (HIV-EM).* Paper presented to the III International Conference on AIDS, Washington, DC.

Siegel, K. (1986). AIDS; The social dimension. *Psychiatric Annals, 16*(3), 168–172.

Siegel, K., Grodsky, P. B., & Herman, A. (1986). AIDS risk-reduction guidelines: A review and analysis. *Journal of Community Health, 11*(4), 233–243.

Siegel, K., Mesagno, F., Chen, J. Y., & Christ, G. (1987, June). *Factors distinguishing homosexual males practicing safe and risky sex.* Paper presented to the III International Conference on AIDS, Washington, DC.

Silver, R., & Wortman, C. (1980). Coping with undesirable life events. In J. Garber & M.

Seligman (Eds.), *Human helplessness: Theory and applications* (pp. 279–373). New York: Academic Press.

Small, C. B., Laper, G., & Ricci, L. (1987, June). *Homelessness in patients with the acquired immune deficiency syndrome (AIDS)*. Paper presented to the III International Conference on AIDS, Washington, DC.

Snider, W., Simpson, D., Nielson, S., Gold, J. W. M., Metroka, C. E., & Posner, J. B. (1983). Neurological complications of acquired immunodeficiency syndrome: Analysis of 50 patients. *Annals of Internal Neurology, 14*, 1413–1418.

Solomon, L. (1986, November). Community interventions for AIDS: Lessons from other health promotion areas. In J. A. Kelly (Chair), *AIDS: The role of behavioral intervention*. Symposium presented to the Annual Meeting of the Association for the Advancement of Behavior Therapy, Chicago.

Solomon, L. J. (in press). Prevention of the spread of AIDS: An interview with Jeffrey A. Kelly. *Journal of Primary Prevention,*

Sonabend, J. A., Witkin, S. S., & Purtilo, D. T. (1985). A multifactorial model for the development of AIDS in homosexual men. *Annals of the New York Academy of Sciences, 437*, 177–183.

Sotheran, J. L., Abdul-Quader, A. S., Friedman, S. R., Des Jarlais, D. C., Marmor, M., & Bartelme, S. (1987, June). *Needle cleaning knowledge among intravenous drug users in treatment and AIDS prevention policy*. Paper presented to the III International Conference on AIDS, Washington, DC.

South, K. T. (undated). *Pastoral care to people with AIDS: A ministry of reconciliation*. Pamphlet available from AIDS Atlanta, 811 Cypress Street, N.E., Atlanta, GA 30348.

Spiegel, D., Bloom, J., & Yalom, I. (1981). Group support for patients with metastatic cancer. *Archives of General Psychiatry, 38*, 527–533.

Stall, R., McKusick, L., Wiley, J., Coates, T. J., & Ostrow, D. G. (1986). Alcohol and drug use during sexual activity and compliance with safe sex guidelines for AIDS: The AIDS behavioral research project. *Health Education Quarterly, 13*(4).

Staquet, J. M., Hemmer, R., and Baert, A. (1986). *AIDS and AIDS-related Complex*. New York: Oxford University Press.

Stempel, R., Moulton, J., Kelly, T., Osmond, D., & Moss, A. R. (1987, June). *Patterns of distress following HIV antibody test notification*. Paper presented to the III International Conference on AIDS, Washington, DC.

Stevens, C. E., Taylor, P. E., Rodriguez, S., & Rubenstein, P. (1987, June). *Recreational drugs and HIV infection: Relationship to risk of infection and immune deficiency*. Paper presented to the III International Conference on AIDS, Washington, DC.

Stevens, C. E., Taylor, P. E., Zang, E. A., Rodriguez de Cordoba, S., & Rubinstein, P. (1987, June). *Incidence of HIV infection in homosexual men in a high risk area: Implications for vaccine trial design*. Paper presented to the III International Conference on AIDS, Washington, DC.

St. Lawrence, J. S., Husfeldt, B. A., Kelly, J. A., Hood, H. V., & Smith, S., Jr. (in press). The stigma of AIDS: Fear of disease and prejudice toward gays. *Journal of Homosexuality,*

Stokes, B. (1982). Self-help in the eighties. *Citizen Participation, 3* 5–7.

Strauss, L. M., Solomon, L. J., Costanza, M. C., Worden, J. K., & Foster, R. S., Jr. (1987). Breast self-examination practices and attitudes of women with and without a history of breast cancer. *Journal of Behavioral Medicine, 10*(4) 337–350.

Stuart, R. B. (1980). *Helping couples change*. New York: Guilford Press.

Swain, M. A., & Stekel, S. B. (1981). Influencing adherence among hypertensives. *Research in Nursing and Health, 4*, 213–222.

Suinn, R. (1977). *Manual: Anxiety management training*. Fort Collins, CO: Rocky Mountain Behavioral Sciences Institute.

Suinn, R. (1980). Behavioral intervention methods for stress and anxiety. In I. Jutash & L. Schlesinger (Eds.), *Handbook on stress and anxiety*. San Francisco: Jossey-Bass.

Suinn, R., & Deffenbacher, J. (1982). The self control of anxiety. In P. Karoly & F. Kanfer (Eds.), *The psychology of self-management: From theory to practice*. New York: Pergamon Press.

Taylor, S. (1983). Adjustment to threatening events: A theory of cognitive adaptation. *American Psychologist, 38,* 1161–1173.

Taylor, S. E., Falke, R. L., Shoptaw, S. J., & Lichtman, R. R. (1986). Social support, support groups, and the cancer patient. *Journal of Consulting and Clinical Psychology, 54,* 608–615.

Taylor, S. E., Lichtman, R. R., Wood, J. V., Bluming, A. Z., Dosak, G. M., & Leibowitz, R. O. (1985). Illness-related and treatment factors in psychological adjustment to breast cancer. *Cancer, 55,* 2506–2513.

Temoshok, L., Sweet, D. M., Moulton, J. M., & Zich, J. (1987, June). *A longitudinal study of distress and coping in men with AIDS and AIDS related complex.* Paper presented to the III International Conference on AIDS, Washington, DC.

Temoshok, L., Sweet, D. M., & Zich, J. (1987). A three city comparison of the public's knowledge and attitudes about AIDS. *Psychology and Health, 1,* 43–60.

Temoshok, L., Zich, T., Solomon, G. F., & Stites, D. P. (1987, June). *An intense psychoimmunologic study of long-surviving persons with AIDS.* Paper presented to the III International Conference on AIDS, Washington, DC.

Tenneriello, L., Callan, M., Gordon, L., Levine, J., Poust, B., & Drucker, E. (1987, June). *A hospital-based volunteer program utilizing methadone patients and others to provide support for inner-city AIDS patients.* Paper presented to the III International Conference on AIDS, Washington, DC.

Thoits, P. A. (1986). Social support as coping assistance. *Journal of Consulting and Clinical Psychology, 54,* 416–423.

Thompson, E. I. (1978). Smoking education programs, 1960–1976. *American Journal of Public Health, 68,* 250–257.

Tillett, G. J. (1987, June). *Anti-discrimination legislation and the reduction of social disruption caused by AIDS.* Paper presented to the III International Conference on AIDS, Washington, DC.

Tross, S. Hirsch, D., Rabkin, B., Berry, C., & Holland, J. C. B. (1987, June). *Determinants of current psychiatric disorder in AIDS spectrum patients.* Paper presented to the III International Conference on AIDS, Washington, DC.

Truax, C. B., & Mitchell, K. M. (1971). Research on certain therapist interpersonal skills in relation to therapy process and outcome. In A. E. Bergin & S. L. Garfield (Eds.), *Handbook of psychotherapy and behavior change.* New York: Wiley.

Truax, C. B., Wargo, D. G., Frank, J. D., Imber, S. D., Battle, C. C., Hoehn-Saric, R., Nash, E. H., & Stone, A. R. (1966). Therapist empathy, genuineness, and warmth and patient therapeutic outcome. *Journal of Consulting Psychology, 320,* 395–401.

Trussell, J., Bloom, D., & Pebley, A. (1981). Correcting contraception failure rates for sample composition and sample selection bias. *Social Biology, 28,* 293–298.

Turner, R. J. (1983). Direct, indirect, and moderating effects of social support on psychological distress and associated conditions. In H. B. Kaplan IEd.), *Psychosocial stress: Trends in theory and research* (pp. 105–155). New York: Academic Press.

United States Department of Health and Human Services. (1986a). *Surgeon general's report on AIDS.* Washington, DC: Author.

United States Department of Health and Human Services. (1986b). Coping with AIDS: Psychological and social considerations in helping people with HTLV-III infection. Rockville, MD: National Institute of Mental Health.

Upper, D., & Cautela, J. R. (1977). *Covert conditioning.* New York: Pergamon Press.

Vachon, M. (1979). *The importance of social support in the longitudinal adaptation to bereavement and breast cancer.* Paper presented to the American Psychological Association, New York.

Van de Perre, P., Rouvroy, D., Lepage, P., Bogaerts, J., Kestelyn, P., Kayihigi, J., Hekker, A. C., Butzler, J. P., & Clumeck, N. (1984). Acquired immunodeficiency syndrome in Rwanda. *Lancet, 2,* 62–65.

Videka-Sherman, L. (1982). Coping with the death of a child: A study over time. *American Journal of Orthopsychiatry, 52,* 688–698.

Vishnubhakat, S. M., Kaplan, M., & Beresford, H. R. (1987, June). *Clinical and electrophysiologi-*

cal features of neuropathy in AIDS. Paper presented to the III International Conference on AIDS, Washington, DC.

Visscher, B., Detels, R., Phair, J., Rinaldo, C., Kaslow, R., & Fox, R. (1987, June). *Reversibility and progression of persisting AIDS-related complex.* Paper presented to the III International Conference on AIDS, Washington, DC.

Voeller, B. (1986). AIDS transmission and saliva. *Lancet, 1,* 1099–1100.

Volberding, P. (1984). Kaposi's sarcoma. In P. Ebbesen, R. S. Biggar, & M. Melbye (Eds.), *AIDS—A basic guide for clinicians* (pp. 99–112). Copenhagen: Munksgaard.

Walker, L. A. (1987). What comforts AIDS families. *The New York Times Magazine,* June 21, pp. 16–23.

Wallace, J. I., Downes, J., Ott, A., Reise, R., Monroe, J., Jordan, D., Thomas, Y., Glickman, E., Rogozinski, L., & Chess, L. (1983). T-cell ratios in New York City prostitutes, *Lancet, 1,* 58.

Wallston, B. S., Alagna, S. W., DeVellis, B. M., & DeVellis, R. E. (1983). Social support and physical health. *Health Psychology, 2,* 367–391.

Walton, R. (1987, June). *AIDS on campus: Strategies for response.* Paper presented to the III International Conference on AIDS, Washington, DC.

Ward, J. W., Deppe, D. A., Samson, S., Perkins, H., Fernando, L., Holland, P., Feorino, P. M., Thompson, P., Kleinman, S., & Allen, J. R. (1987). Risk of human immunodeficiency virus infection from blood donors who later developed the acquired immunodeficiency syndrome. *Annals of Internal Medicine, 106,* 61–62.

Watters, J. K. (1987, June). *Preventing human immunodeficiency virus contagion among intravenous drug users: The impact of street-based education on risk-behavior.* Paper presented to the III International Conference on AIDS, Washington, DC.

Weber, J. N., Wadsworth, J., Rogers, L. A., Moshitael, O., Scott, K., McManus, T., Berrie, E., Jeffries, D. J., Harris, J. R., & Pinching, A. J. (1986). Three-year prospective study of HTLV-III/LAV infection in homosexual men. *Lancet, 1,* 1179–1182.

Weisman, A. D., & Worden, J. W. (1975). Psychological analysis of cancer deaths. *Omega, 6,* 61–75.

Williams, A. E., Kleinman, S., Lamberson, H., Popovsky, M., Williams, K., & Dodd, R. (1987, June). *Assessment of the demographic and motivational characteristics of HIV seropositive blood donors.* Paper presented to the III International Conference on AIDS, Washington, DC.

Willoughby, B., Schechter, M. T., Boyko, W. J., Craib, K. J. P., Weaver, M. S., & Douglas, B. (1987, June). *Sexual practices and condom use in a cohort of homosexual men. Evidence of differential modification between seropositive and seronegative men.* Paper presented to the III International Conference on AIDS, Washington, DC.

Wodak, A. D., Dolan, K. Imrie, A., Gold, J., Whyte, B. M., & Cooper, D. A. (1987, June). *HIV antibodies in needles and syringes used by intravenous drug users.* Paper presented to the III International Conference on AIDS, Washington, DC.

Wolcott, D. L. (1986a). Psychosocial aspects of acquired immune deficiency syndrome and the primary care physician. *Annals of Allergy, 57,* 98–102.

Wolcott, D. L. (1986b). Neuropsychiatric syndromes in AIDS and AIDS-related diseases. In L. McKusick (Ed.), (pp. 46–62). *What to do about AIDS: Physicians and mental health professionals discuss the issues.* Berkeley: University of California Press.

Wolfred, T., Dunne, R., & Peabody, J. (1987, June). *Developing community based service organizations.* Roundtable discussion, III International Conference on AIDS, Washington, DC.

Wolpe, J. (1982). *The practice of behavior therapy.* New York: Pergamon Press.

Worden, J. K., Flynn, B. S., Solomon, L. J., Costanzo, M. C., Foster, R. S., Jr., Dorwalt, A. L., Driscoll, M. A., & Askikaga, T. (1987). A community-wide breast self-exam education program. In P. Engstrom (Ed.), *Advances in cancer control IV: The war on cancer—15 years of progress.*

World Health Organization. (1987, March). *Special programme on AIDS: Strategies and structure projected needs.*

Wright, M. M. (1987, June). *A survey of residency programs for persons with AIDS.* Paper presented to the III International Conference on AIDS, Washgton, DC.

Yarchoan, R., Berg, G., Brouwers, P., Fischl, M. A., Spitzer, A. R., Wichman, A., Grafman, J., Thomas, R. V., Safai, B., Brunetti, A., Perno, C. F., Schmidt, P. J., Larson, S. M., Myers, C. E., & Broder, S. (1987). Response of human immunodeficiency virus associated neurological disease to 3'azido-3'-deozythymidine. *Lancet, 1,* 132–135.

Yarchoan, R., & Broder, S. (1987). Development of antiretroviral therapy for the acquired immunodeficiency syndrome and related disorders. A progress report. *New England Journal of Medicine, 316,* 557–564.

Young, E. W. D. (1986). AIDS: Emerging moral questions. *Journal of American College Health, 34*(5), 240–242.

Young, G. P., Van der Weyden, M. B., Rose, I. S., & Dudley, F. J. (1979). Lymphopenic and lymphocyte transformation in alcoholics. *Experientia, 35,* 268–269.

Ziegler, J. L., & Abrams, D. I. (1985). The AIDS-related complex. In V. T. DeVita, S. Helman, & S. A. Rosenberg (Eds.), *AIDS: Etiology, diagnosis, treatment, and prevention.* New York: J. B. Lippincott.

Zones, J. S., Beeson, D. R., Echenberg, D. F., Rutherford, G. W., & O'Malley, P. O. (1987, June). *Management of confidentiality by a cohort of gay and bisexual men who have learned their antibody status.* Paper presented to the III International Conference on AIDS, Washington, DC.

Zuckerman, M., Tushup, R., & Finner, S. (1976). Sexual attitudes and experience: Attitude and personality correlates and changes produced by a course on sexuality. *Journal of Consulting and Clinical Psychology, 144,* 7–19.

Index